Making
WINE
with
Fruits, Roots
& Flowers

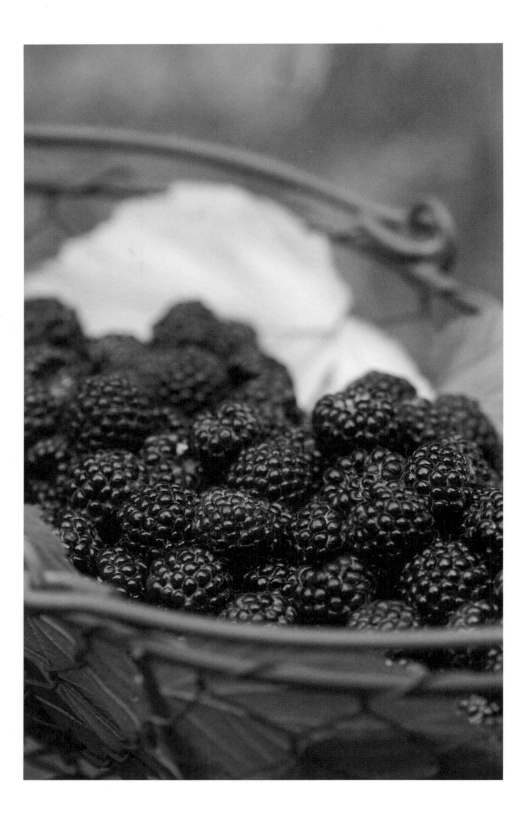

Making
WINE
with
Fruits, Roots
& Flowers

Recipes for Distinctive & Delicious Wild Wines

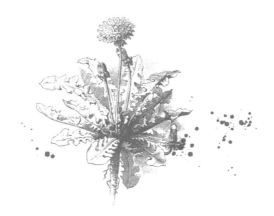

MARGARET CROWTHER

BETTERWAY HOME

First published in the US in 2012 by
F+W Media Inc.
10150 Carver Road, Cincinnati,
Ohio 45242, US

ISBN 978-1-4403-2034-7

1 3 5 7 9 10 8 6 4 2

PRODUCED BY
Fine Folio Publishing Limited
6 Bourne Terrace, Bourne Hill, Wherstead,
Ipswich, Suffolk, IP2 8NG, UK
www.finefoliopublishing.com

DESIGNER
Glyn Bridgewater

ILLUSTRATOR
Coral Mula

EDITOR
Alison Copland

Printed and bound by
Voion Printing Group (International) Co., Ltd
Unit 305–306, 3rd Floor, Yen Sheng Centre,
64 Hoi Yuen Road, Kwun Tong, KLN, Hong Kong

CONTENTS

GOOD WINE
IS A GOOD FAMILIAR CREATURE
IF IT BE WELL USED

OTHELLO, WILLIAM SHAKESPEARE

INTRODUCTION

Officially, by strict definition, wine has to be the product of the grape. But tradition has always used the term more widely to encompass the fermented juices of fruits, flowers and vegetables – wild, country wines. In theory, wine from grapes involves nothing but the fruits themselves. Grapes have the sugars, yeasts, and balanced acids required to turn their juices into palatable wine. Meanwhile, other fruits, vegetables, and especially flowers lack either natural sugars, the right yeasts and acids, or sufficient juices to be converted into alcoholic drinks without the addition of water, wine yeast, acids, and usually sugar for the yeast to work on.

In fact, however, ever since the days of Pasteur, the wine produced commercially from grapes has been less than completely 'natural', involving procedures whereby the natural yeasts on the fruits are replaced with perfected yeast strains, and many other tinkering and sterilizing interventions. We need make no apology for calling our own wild or country wines by that name, in the old and honourable tradition. Remember, sparkling Gooseberry wine was often passed off as Champagne, even in France, and grape wines were frequently 'adulterated' with Elderberry wine to improve them until the recent past.

Country wines contain and preserve the true essence of their original ingredients, and whether we drink them at the table with our food or – which I prefer – as special drinks that can stand up in their own right, nothing can compare to the pleasure of slowly sipping clear, beautifully tinted wild wines, and sharing them with friends.

Each sip reminds you of the day you picked the fruit, the pleasures of mixing and mashing, fermenting and bottling, the spring day, the summer heat, the autumn bounty. Each sip is a just reward for your pleasant efforts.

Country people used to make wines, cordials, sweet syrups, and other drinks as a way of preserving garden produce and wild fruits and flowers while providing household remedies and tonics, and, of course, for the pure pleasure of drinking them. We cannot suppose they studied the science of this occupation, but then this was a traditional country pursuit and they had other people to learn from and to rely on for encouragement. They would have observed the procedures taking place as they were growing up, and when in doubt could ask advice from family and neighbors.

Somewhere along the line, that tradition has been broken. Nowadays, as winemakers, we are often starting from scratch and will probably need to do a bit of fast-tracking to make up for lost experience. The trial and error approach can make for a long learning process, and so many failures are easily avoided with a minimal knowledge of what is involved.

The best short-cut to perfection is to have a little understanding of the method and science involved in making wines from things we grow or gather from the wild before we begin. This part of the book aims to give a very brief account of what is involved, and what can go wrong, to set your home winemaking off on the right track.

IN VINO VERITAS
(TRUTH COMES OUT IN WINE)
PLINY THE ELDER (AD 23–79), ROMAN SCHOLAR

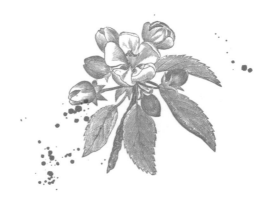

ABOUT WINEMAKING

Winemaking is a perfectible skill, and most people find it includes an encouraging amount of beginner's luck, which gets it off to a satisfyingly good start. The best part of it is that it is an absorbing – yet not very time-consuming – hobby, and also an inexpensive one, involving only a small amount of equipment and free or low-cost ingredients. Certainly, much patience is required: for example, many wines are not ready for bottling until at least six months after the day you started them, and then some of them need to be allowed to mature for two years or even more before they yield of their delicious best. During this time, however, you need to do little more than check on their progress once in a while, and look forward to drinking them.

Wines in the make do need personal attention and may sulk if they are left unattended in a corner. Yet the amount of daily time you need to spend on them is minimal, while the pleasure you will get in selecting and preparing the ingredients and starting off the procedure, listening to the energetic fizz of open fermenting and the contented steady plop of bubbles escaping through the airlock of a demijohn filled with promise, watching a cloudy, sweet liquid gradually turn into a clear, alcoholic one, and finally getting the finished wild wine to trickle into freshly cleaned and waiting bottles, is a more than ample reward for the simple labors you expended – and a homely pleasure that is very hard to beat.

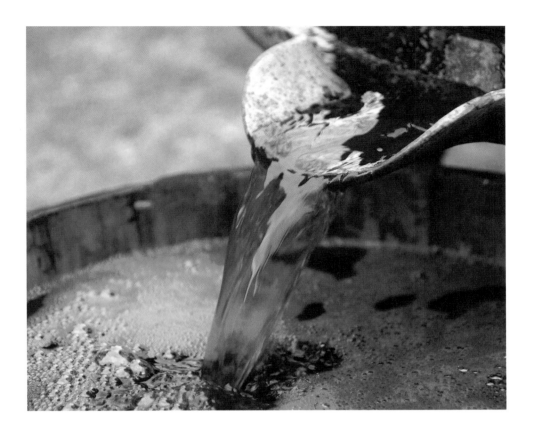

You will need somewhere warm and draft-free to store the wine-to-be for a week or so at the stage when you are extracting juices and flavor and getting fermentation going (such as a corner of the kitchen); a room or cupboard in which you can store a jar or more of fermenting wine undisturbed at a constant temperature of about 16°C (60°F) for up to a year (cool for a room, by modern standards, yet not cold); somewhere cooler to keep the maturing wine in the bottle (a cellar is of course ideal, but an unheated cupboard or spare room will be fine), and also a certain amount of equipment, some of which will already be to hand in the kitchen.

Skill is involved, perhaps even art, but the business of home winemaking is really not very demanding. So next time you take a country walk, be on the lookout for wild ingredients; if you don't know what to do with an unexpectedly large crop of apples or pears, or if someone gives you an overwhelming quantity of homegrown runner beans, remember that they can all be used for wine.

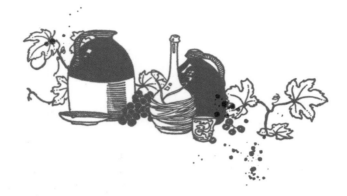

EQUIPMENT

Most of the essential equipment for winemaking can be bought new at very reasonable cost, and may even be found second-hand in charity shops, car boot or garage sales, and similar haunts. A good deal of what you need can be improvised or is already in your kitchen. All you will really need is listed below, in the order in which you will need it, together with other things that might be helpful, and extra gadgets – modestly priced – that may not be essential but that can make winemaking go more smoothly. Why you will need it, and what you will do with it, will all be made clear in the 'Getting Started' section (see page 27).

You will need

Large bucket with lid or cover (often called a 'bin') for steeping/fermenting
* should be food-grade plastic and ideally marked on the inside with volumes
* purpose-made bins are readily available from suppliers
* a 10-liter (2-gallon) version is needed for the recipes in this book, to allow room for steeping the ingredients plus headroom during the vigorous fermentation stage
* an open bucket can be used, and covered with a clean cloth or sheet of plastic tied round the rim

ESSENTIAL EQUIPMENT

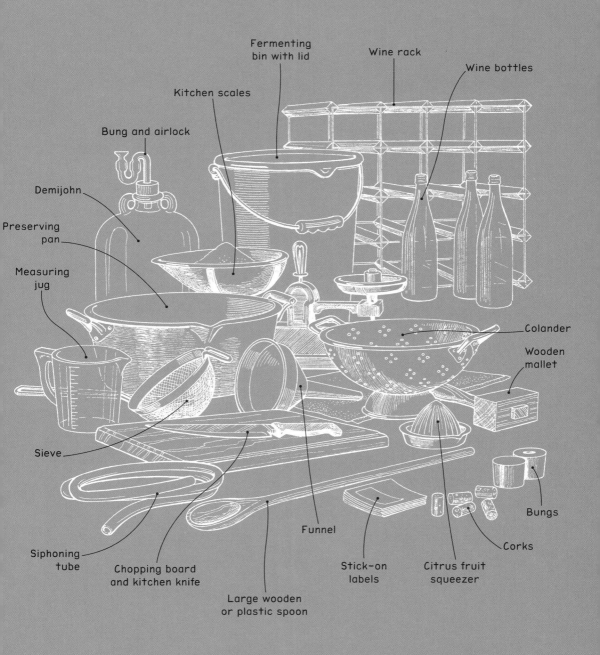

Fermenting bin with lid

Wine rack

Wine bottles

Kitchen scales

Bung and airlock

Demijohn

Preserving pan

Measuring jug

Colander

Wooden mallet

Sieve

Bungs

Siphoning tube

Chopping board and kitchen knife

Funnel

Stick-on labels

Citrus fruit squeezer

Corks

Large wooden or plastic spoon

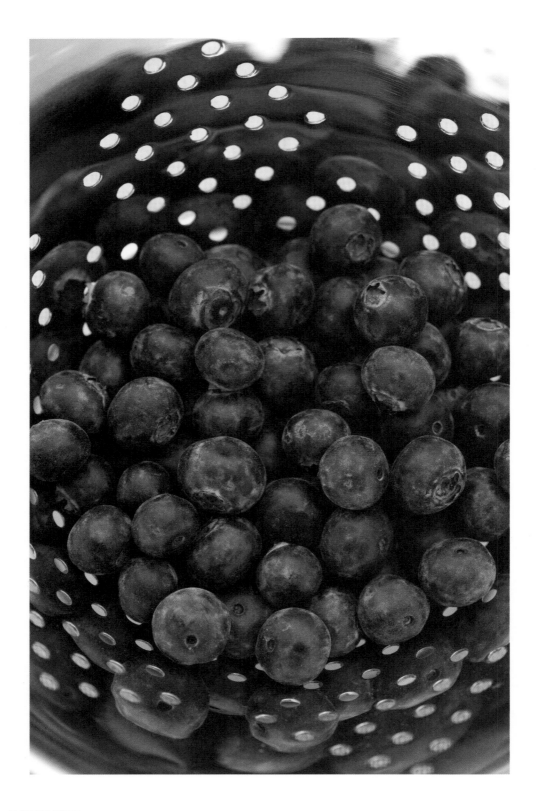

Kitchen scales for weighing ingredients
* the maximum weight required for these wines is usually about 3 kg (7 lb)

Large chopping board and kitchen knife
* kitchen scissors can also sometimes be helpful, especially with flower wines

Measuring jug for water and fruit juice, and for some dry ingredients that are measured by volume
* these are available from specialist suppliers, but an ordinary glass or plastic kitchen jug will be fine

Preserving pan or very large saucepan for ingredients that have to be boiled
* this should be made from stainless steel or unchipped enamel-ware – not copper, iron, or brass

Ordinary kitchen colander or large sieve for washing fruit, flowers, and leaves
* a very large sieve will also be useful for straining off liquids after steeping or boiling

Wooden mallet, meat tenderizer, or rolling pin for crushing fruit and softened vegetables
* any wooden implement should be very carefully cleaned and sterilized
* a potato masher can be useful for crushing cooked vegetables
* the base of a large, super-clean glass jar can be used for crushing soft summer fruit such as raspberries, strawberries, and blackcurrants

Ordinary citrus fruit squeezer and zester (parer) for the many recipes that use citrus fruit

Large wooden or purpose-made plastic spoon for stirring
* the longer the better, so that it will reach right to the bottom of the bin
* special stirring paddles are available, which can be useful for heavyweight ingredients or larger quantities

Glass demijohn (wine-jar)
* this is a now-traditional heavy glass jar with lugs and a narrow mouth. The opening will be fitted with a bung and airlock for the closed fermentation stage and bunged up completely if you wish to mature the wine in bulk before bottling
* the recipes in this book are for a standard 4.5-liter (1-gallon) jar
* a spare jar will be useful and will help to simplify operations with many recipes
* a dark jar is useful for recipes where the wine needs to be protected from light, but is not essential
* plastic demijohns are available from specialist suppliers, with the stated advantage that they have a drilled cap and rubber grommet into which the airlock can easily be inserted for a good fit, and of course that they are unbreakable

Purpose-made bung and airlock (various types of airlock are available, in glass or plastic) to fit into the demijohn during the closed fermentation process

Purpose-made bung to stop up the demijohn when the wine is being matured
* a cunning little safety bung is available, which stops air from entering, but which will allow any excess gases to be released from the jar, insuring against possible explosions from imprisoned, still-fermenting wine

Large funnel (food-grade plastic, stainless steel, or enamel-ware) and **straining cloths**, including fine cloths for when very fine particles need to be strained out

Length of flexible food-grade plastic or rubber siphoning tube for racking the wine, transferring the wine from jar to jar, and bottling
* 2 m (6½ ft) is the normal length

Glass wine bottles, ideally including one or two half-bottles
* used bottles are fine, as long as they are perfectly clean
* Champagne bottles, in extra-strong glass with indented bases, are essential for sparkling wine

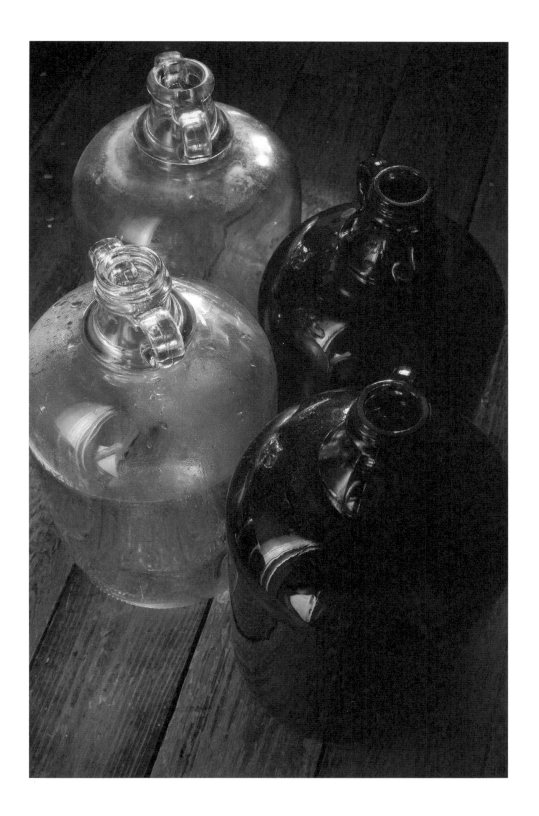

Purpose-made corks
* these must be new – various cork and plastic 'corks' are available, including plastic 'Champagne corks' and wires (called 'cages') that are essential for sparkling wine

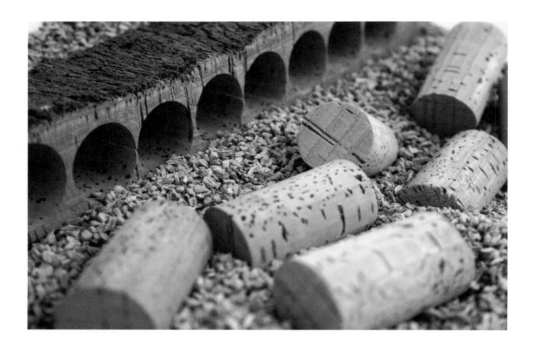

Stick-on labels (for labeling the bottles)

Wine rack for storing the finished wines
* wine racks can often be found second-hand

The following may also help

Mincer – useful for some ingredients, including dried fruit, but not essential

Large glass or glazed china/earthenware kitchen bowl – can be useful for initial preparation/steeping of some ingredients before they are put into a fermenting bin
* you will also need a clean kitchen cloth or plastic film to cover the bowl

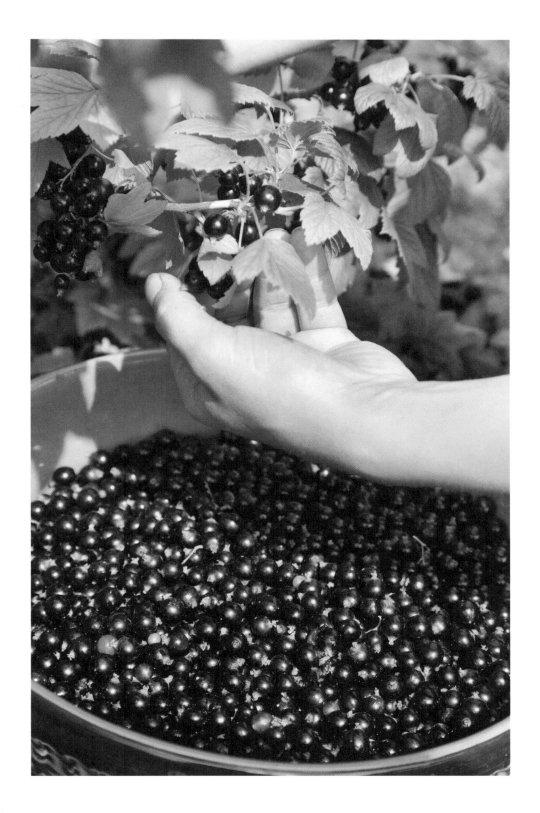

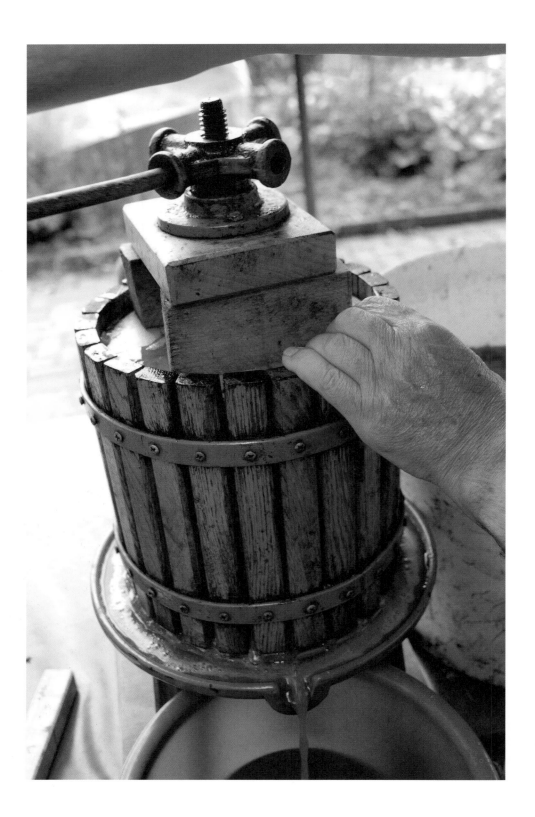

Fermenting mat (also called 'heating pad,' 'heating belt,' or 'heating tray')
* these are electrically heated pads on which to stand the jar of fermenting wine to keep it at the correct temperature during fermentation

Proper fruit press (for crushing hard raw ingredients such as apples)
* this would be a luxury, but ideal if you need to prepare large quantities

Purpose-made pulper (for pulping fruit and vegetable ingredients)
* these are fitted to an electric drill for use by macho winemakers

Hydrometer
* this is a device for measuring specific gravity (now properly called 'relative gravity'), enabling you to measure the sugar content/alcohol level in a sample of liquid at different stages and check the progress of the wine. Hydrometers usually come complete with a test jar to hold the sample
* a cheap and useful gadget known as a 'vinometer' is available from some suppliers. This takes a sample of the wine into a tube and shows the level of alcohol present

pH test strips
* acid test papers to check the acidity or otherwise of ingredients. Your own taste buds can be a fairly good guide

Autosiphon
* this is a gadget that takes the sucking out of siphoning. With a controllable piston, it will siphon right to the bottom of the liquid and helps to avoid sucking up the solid deposit at the bottom of the wine jar (see page 39)
* a very optional extra, but inexpensive and worth considering, especially if you become a regular winemaker

Thermometer for accurately taking the temperature of infusions and musts (wine in the making)
* a jam-making kitchen thermometer is fine, as is the finger test, but specialized thermometers are available that hang inside the winemaking container

HELPFUL EQUIPMENT

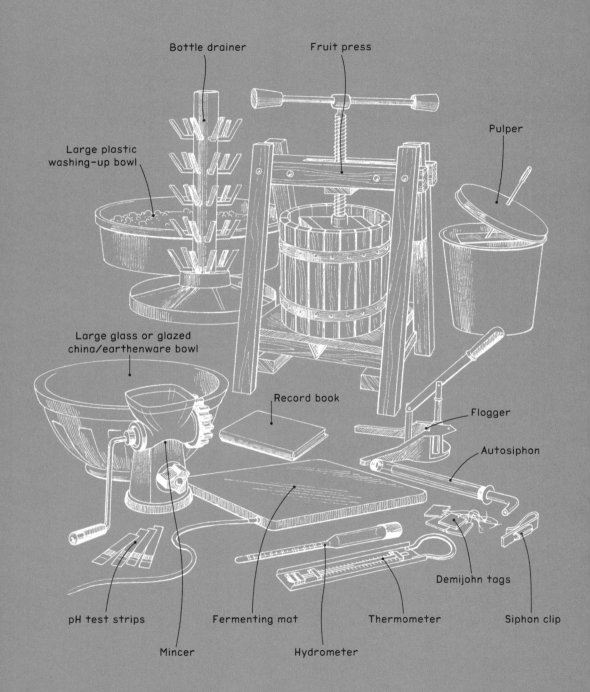

Bottle drainer

Fruit press

Pulper

Large plastic washing-up bowl

Large glass or glazed china/earthenware bowl

Record book

Flogger

Autosiphon

pH test strips

Mincer

Fermenting mat

Hydrometer

Thermometer

Demijohn tags

Siphon clip

Siphon clip
* a small device, sold at a small price, that helpfully holds your tubing in place while you are fiddling with the other end when siphoning wine from container to container and into bottles
* this could be described as an inessential necessity that will save a lot of frustration

Large plastic washing-up bowl to hold up to eight bottles
* this will catch any spills that are bound to occur during bottling; alternatively, layers of newspapers can be used

Flogger
* this is a mechanical aid to corking; various types are available from suppliers

Bottle drainer
* this holds sterilized bottles upside down in an orderly way and enables them to drain neatly

Demijohn tags for labeling the filled demijohns
* a proper labeling system makes you feel much better organized

Record book
* keeping track of what you did and when you did it in a record book will be vital so that you know how to repeat your successes and learn from your mistakes

For preparation and cleaning of equipment

Bottle brush
* this should be long enough to reach right to the base of the bottles, and have a bristly end so that it cleans thoroughly

Cranked brush for thoroughly cleaning demijohns
* this enables the 'shoulders' of the jar to be properly cleaned

Tiny brushes for cleaning inside the airlock

PREPARATION AND CLEANING EQUIPMENT

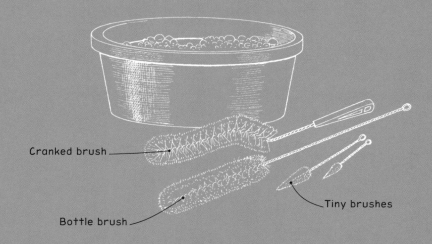

Cranked brush

Tiny brushes

Bottle brush

TRADITIONAL ALTERNATIVES AND OTHER EQUIPMENT

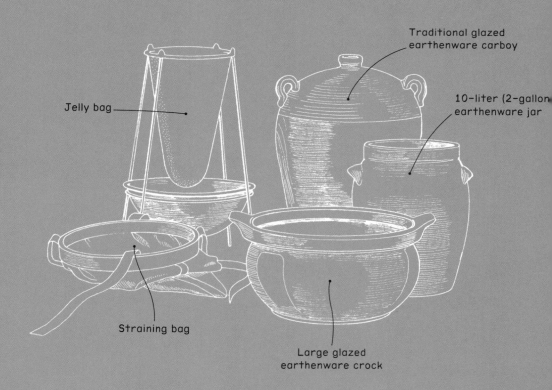

Jelly bag

Traditional glazed
earthenware carboy

10-liter (2-gallon)
earthenware jar

Straining bag

Large glazed
earthenware crock

Traditional alternatives and other equipment

Very large straining bag

* using a very large, strong straining bag which fits inside the fermenting bin enables you to remove and drain the pulp from the liquid with minimum fuss, but it does make stirring more complicated

Jelly bag

* this is useful in some recipes, where squeezing the fruit could cause the wine to go cloudy

Large glazed earthenware crock

* a crock is a wide-topped heavy-based bowl, glazed on the inside, also used in the past for breadmaking. If you use a traditional crock for steeping/open fermenting, make sure that it is not cracked or chipped

10-liter (2-gallon) earthenware jar

* the traditional cylindrical open-topped jar for open-fermenting can still be used as long as it is in good condition, but the top must be covered with several layers of fine muslin or kitchen film

Traditional glazed earthenware carboy

* a heavy jar with a narrow opening at the top, used as a demijohn for closed fermenting and storing. It is less than ideal for fermenting, since you cannot see what is going on inside it, and are unlikely to get an airlock bung to fit it, but – properly bunged or stoppered – it would be perfect for maturing and storing wine as it keeps out the light, and maintains a constant temperature well

---

WARNING

If using traditional glazed jars, make sure they are salt-glazed, not lead-glazed. Salt glazes look thin and hard and give off a sharp note when struck. Lead glazes have a soft, honey-colored appearance and sound dull when tapped.

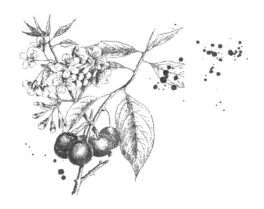

RANGE OF WINES

Winemaking can be a year-round activity, with some fresh ingredient available at just about every season, since almost anything that grows can be turned to wine. From early spring there are the many wild flowers, with Agrimony, Gorse, and Clover taking over when Coltsfoot and Dandelion are in short supply. Early summer supplies May Blossom (Hawthorn Blossom) and Elderflowers, and then the fruits begin to appear. The soft fruits come first, with Black- and Redcurrants, then summer Cherries, Gooseberries, and soon Raspberries and Loganberries. Late summer produces a wild harvest of Blackberries, Elderberries, and the hedgerow fruits of Hawthorn, while Mulberries are ripening in gardens.

Meanwhile the vegetable garden has been producing Rhubarb and Peas, and Runner Beans are getting into their stride with Parsley and Marigolds flourishing, while orchards and fields are yielding new season's Apples, and the various forms of Plums. Then as Pears and later Apples ripen, so the hedgerows are showing Crab Apples, Damsons, and the red Rosehips and blue Sloes that need to be left on the bushes until the frosts. Root vegetables take their turn in winter, and are often best left until the colder weather takes hold.

With citrus fruit, root Ginger, and Bananas among the crop available at low cost all year, plentiful imported summer Apricots and late-summer Peaches and a wealth of frozen summer fruits, dried Apricots, Bananas, vine fruits, and even dried flowers and hedgerow fruit available from herbalists and winemaking suppliers, there is never a shortage of material for homemade wines.

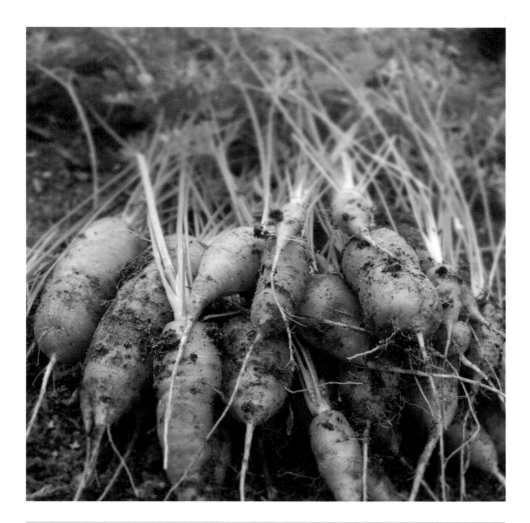

WARNING

Share your homemade wines generously with family and friends, but remember that it is illegal to sell them in any circumstances – even for charity.

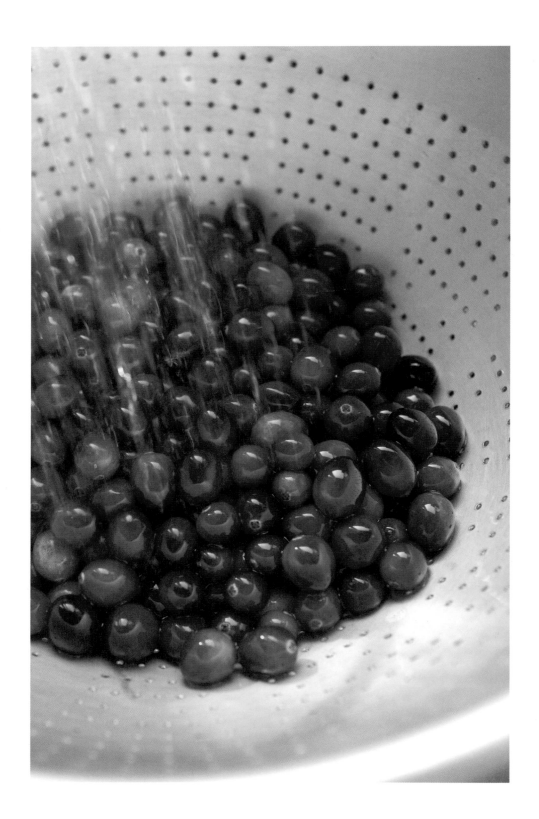

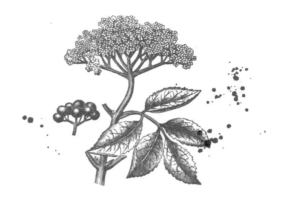

GETTING STARTED

Before you start, the following summary of the basic method outlines what you are going to be doing. It presupposes that you use freshly harvested ingredients (freshly picked fruit can be frozen in suitable quantities for later use) and that they are clean and sound. Every piece of equipment, including fermenting bins, lids, and containers, must be scrupulously clean too, to deter the myriad of bacteria and microscopic fungi that are invisibly swarming about in the air and waiting to invade. Wash equipment in hot water then rinse it in sterilizing solution (available from suppliers) in the kitchen sink, or in the fermenting bin itself, or soak small items in a bowl of sterilizing solution before each use.

Summary of basic method

1   Prepare the fruit, flowers, or vegetables and put them into a large container or fermenting bin. A crushed Campden tablet (see page 38) may be added at this stage. The recipes in this book specify the preparation method in more detail.

Tip Lining the bin with a very large straining bag can make the next steps easier.

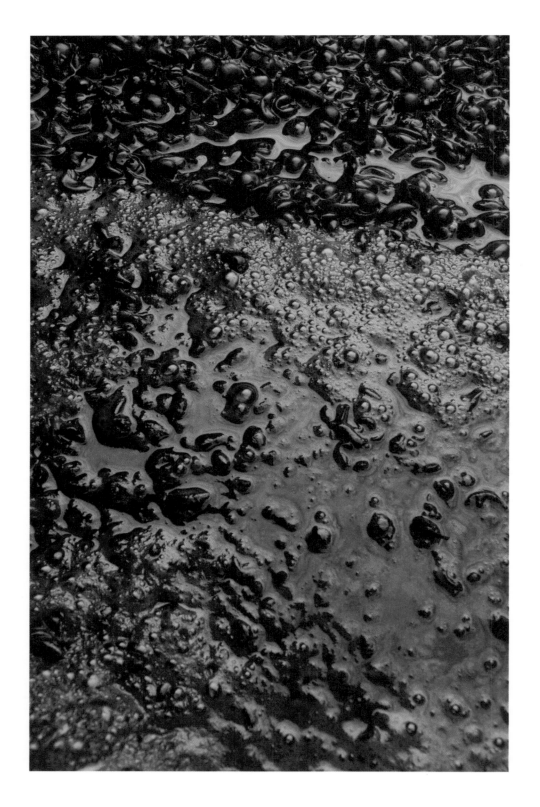

2   Add water and sugar and any other recipe ingredients, stir well, add yeast and nutrient, cover, and leave in a warm place (at 18–24°C/65–75°F) to ferment for up to a week, stirring once or twice a day. (This is the open fermentation stage.)

Adding yeast   If using a Campden tablet, allow 24 hours before adding yeast. If using boiling water, let it cool to 27°C (80°F) or below.

3   Using a jug and straining funnel, strain into a clean jar (demijohn). Top up with boiled but cooled water to just below the jar neck; alternatively, keep any spare liquid in a closed container to use later for topping up.

4   Fit a bung and airlock, fill the airlock reservoir with sterilizing solution, and leave at a constant temperature of around 16°C (60°F) to ferment (the closed fermentation stage). This takes up to three months and often even more. Bubbles of gas will escape through the airlock during this time.

5   Siphon off the liquid (the must) as a sediment (the lees) forms in the jar (called racking), transfer it to a clean jar, top up, and continue fermenting as before. Make sure you do not suck up any of the sediment when siphoning. Repeat as necessary.

6   When there is no more bubbling, and the wine is clear, fermentation has finished. Move the jar to a warmer place for three days to make quite sure that there is no more bubbling.

Hydrometer   If you wish, you can check by taking a hydrometer reading. If it remains the same for three days, the wine is ready.

7   Optional stage: Siphon the wine off the sediment into a clean jar, insert a bung and leave in a cool place to clear and mature. Siphoning will also air the wine to help out any remaining gases.

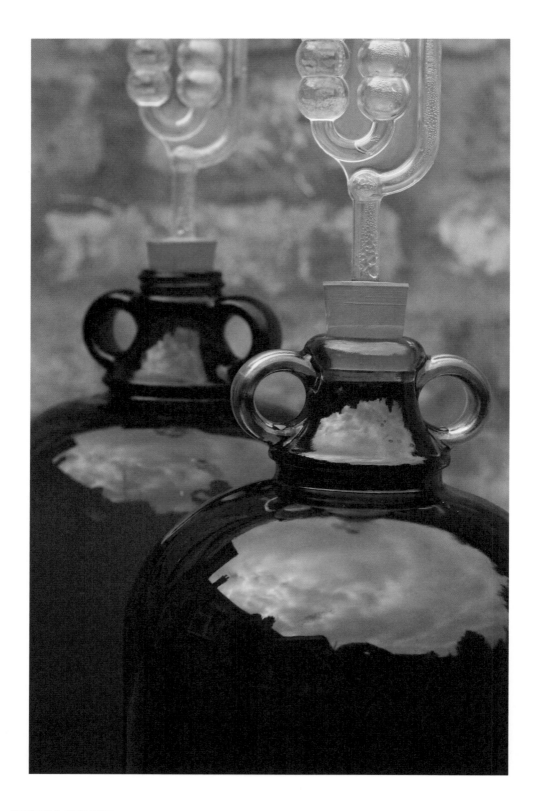

Fining and filtering Add finings now (follow the manufacturer's instructions) if the wine is still cloudy. Wine can also be filtered to make it even clearer.

8   Sterilize the bottles and corks by soaking for 15–30 minutes in sterilizing solution. No need to rinse the bottles before using them.

Stabilizing Stabilize the wine at this point, if required – add one stabilizer tablet (potassium sorbate) and one Campden tablet (sodium metabisulfite), used together. The recipe will state when this is necessary, though some people do it as a precaution with any wine to prevent oxidation, contamination, and in-bottle fermentation. Alternatively, vitamin C may be used to prevent oxidation.

9   Carefully siphon the clear wine into the clean bottles and fit corks. Drive the corks well home and label the bottles.

10 Store the bottles in a cool, dark place for the specified time. Keep them upright for the first week as a precaution (in case fermentation restarts in the bottles), then lay them on their sides. Bottles containing sparkling wine should always be kept upright.

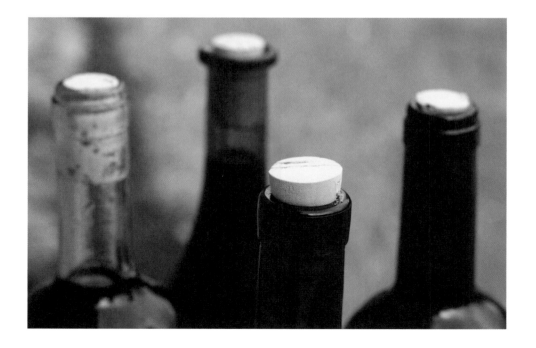

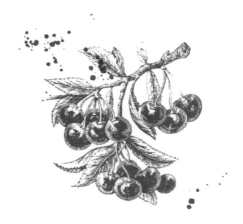

INGREDIENTS AND TECHNIQUES

Country wines and wild wines can be made from just about anything from the vegetable kingdom, but the recipes in this book stick to tradition and use only plant ingredients that have been tried and tested, and enjoyed, over several generations. Additional ingredients are few and simple in nature, and are listed in the order in which they will be needed. Some of the techniques that may not seem obvious are also described, again in the order in which you will need to know about them. These ingredients, and the techniques you use, will all affect the finished wine (see also 'Troubleshooting,' page 48).

Water

Very few country ingredients supply enough juice for wine on their own, so water is added to the main ingredient. Steeping or boiling in water also enables all the flavors and juices to be captured. Old recipes would specify spring water, but it really is not necessary to buy expensive mineral water to make wine. Household tap water is fine. If your tap water is 'chalky,' and you don't already use a water filter jug, it would be a good idea to get one and filter the water before using it. The same applies if your tap water has a 'chemical' taste. Some people also prefer to boil the water for the recipe and allow it to cool before using it.

Steeping Steeping ingredients need to be stirred occasionally to aerate them, but the container should be covered, either with a well-fitting lid or kitchen film or with a clean tea towel secured in place.

Chlorine in the water Many of the recipes in this book specify the use of Campden tablets to guard against contamination by wild yeasts and bacteria (see page 38). A beneficial side-effect of Campden tablets is that they neutralize chlorine, so that their use will also take away the 'chemical' taste of tap water.

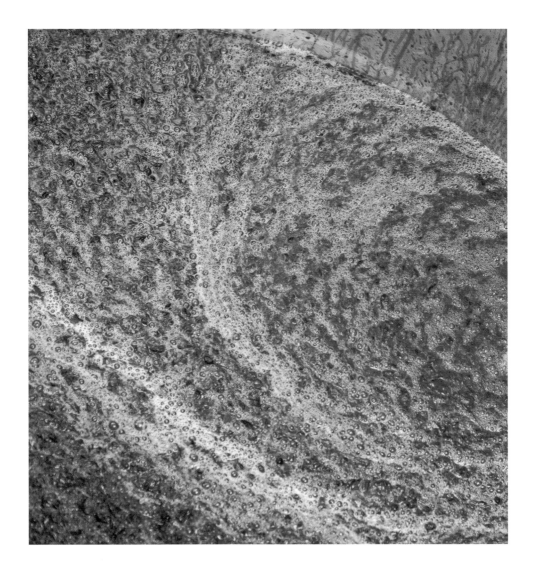

Sugar

Alcohol is produced as the happy result of the action of yeast on sugar. Fruits, and even vegetables, contain their own sugars to varying degrees and a few traditional recipes rely on the sweetness of the main ingredient alone. However, with the exception of grapes, this method is unreliable, and all the recipes here depend on sugar being used. Sugar, in the form of loaf sugar, has been used for many hundreds of years, though honey was a more commonplace form of sweetening in ordinary households.

These recipes normally use ordinary white granulated sugar, though Demerara sugar (raw brown sugar) is sometimes preferred for its special flavor. Demerara sugar is mentioned by name when it is required, and where the recipe ingredients specify 'sugar' the ordinary white sugar is what is meant.

Stirring It is important to make sure that all the sugar is dissolved. Stir thoroughly, especially when cold water is being used. Sugar can be added in the form of ready-dissolved syrup if you prefer (see below). A supply of this syrup is useful for topping up the demijohn after racking.

Making syrup Syrup is made in the ratio of roughly two to one sugar to water, heated and stirred together in a pan then cooled (for example, 1 kg/2 lb sugar and 600 ml/1 pint water). The resulting syrup can be diluted with a little more water.

Yeast

Many old recipes relied on the natural yeasts that flourish on the skins of fruits, and that float about in the wild looking for something to attach themselves to. Otherwise, baker's yeast, which was commonly available, was spread on a piece of toast and this was floated on the surface of the brew. Brewer's yeast was also used indiscriminately in homemade wines. These methods are all very haphazard, and don't achieve the refined results we are aiming for, so modern winemakers use specially prepared yeasts. Various specialized types are available, but unless the recipes specify otherwise the yeast to be used is all-purpose, ready-to-use wine yeast, with nutrient incorporated.

Yeast nutrient or energizer

Yeast is a microscopic form of plant life, and as a living organism it thrives on the right nutrients. Yeast nutrient (sometimes called yeast energizer) supplies beneficial mineral salts and vitamins – chiefly di-ammonium phosphate and vitamin B – to energize and feed the yeast, ensuring that fermentation works effectively. The simplest way to use it is in a combined form of all-purpose yeast and nutrient, but nutrient can be added separately if you prefer. Unless otherwise stated, a combined yeast and nutrient is used in all the recipes in this book.

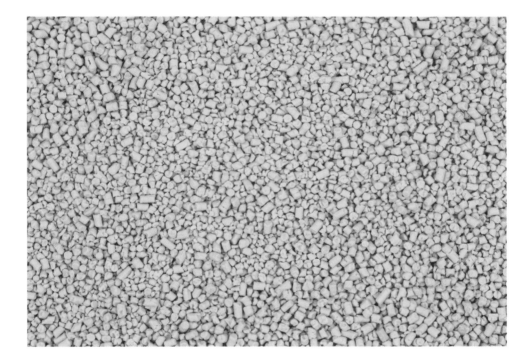

Activating yeast Yeast can be slow to get working in country wines. To get it off to a sure start, you can activate a starter by mixing the yeast with an equal amount of sugar in a cup of warm water (at about 27–30°C/80–86°F, or as stated in the instructions on the sachet). Leave this to stand in a warm place for about 15 minutes until it becomes frothy, and then add it to the fermenting bin.

The action of yeast

Open fermentation Yeast needs not only nutrients but also the right conditions in which to grow. During the open fermentation stage (Step 2), its main desire is for air (oxygen) and warmth, so it needs to be kept at a temperature of 18–24°C (65–75°F), and the ingredients must be well stirred once or twice daily to admit plenty of air. At this stage you are encouraging the yeast to multiply as rapidly as possible. Fermentation is busy and vigorous as the yeast gets to work. The fruit or vegetable pulp will keep on rising to the surface during all this activity (called the cap), and it is best to weigh it down with a scrupulously clean plate as well as keeping the vessel covered. Leave it fermenting away in a warm place for four to five days (or up to a week).

Closed fermentation During closed fermentation (Steps 4 and 5), you will be forcing the yeast to produce alcohol. It now requires less warmth and should be kept at a constant temperature of about 16°C (60°F). With the container closed so that air cannot enter, it gets to work on the sugars present in the liquid and converts them into a mixture of mainly alcohol and carbon dioxide gas. The alcohol is retained in the liquid, while the gas escapes by forcing itself through the airlock, and in doing so it makes a pleasant plopping sound as bubble after bubble of the gas passes into the air. Each yeast cell is capable of reproducing itself many times, and bit by bit exhausted cells sink to the bottom of the jar, forming a deposit known as the lees, while new cells continue the activity. The more the yeast 'works,' the more alcohol is formed.

Sweet or dry wines Either the yeast will continue 'working' until it has consumed just about all the sugar and the resulting wine will be dry, or it will become exhausted before all the sugar is used, and the wine will be sweeter (this will partly depend on the amount of sugar used and the sweetness of the original ingredients).

Pectic enzyme

This generally comes in powder form (well-known names are Pectolase and Super Enzyme) and is an enzyme that breaks down pectins in the natural ingredients. Pectins are found particularly in some fruit, and while they are a boon to jam makers because they help the jam to thicken and set, they are unwelcome in winemaking as they can cause the wine to be cloudy. Pectic enzyme also helps to extract all the juices and flavors of the main ingredients and improves the clarity of the wine, and including it in the ingredients can never do any harm. It is generally best added to warm (not hot) ingredients.

Using your freezer Fruit from the freezer is perfect for wine as the freezing process causes the cell walls to break down, which reduces pectin and encourages the optimum juices and flavor out of the fruit. So don't worry if you cannot use fruit produce on the day you picked it. Just clean it, remove it from its stems or hulls, bag it in recipe-ready quantities, label (of course), and freeze it until you are ready to make wine.

Acid blend

Tannin (tannic acid) and other naturally occurring acids aid the activity of the yeast, help to prevent bacterial contamination, and give body, character, and stability to the finished wine. The acids in 'wild' ingredients often need to be boosted or rebalanced, and acid blend provides a balanced mix supplying tartaric, tannic, citric, and malic acids. Acid blend is not needed in every case, depending on the nature of the main ingredient (see individual recipes), while with certain wild ingredients additional tannin or citric acid is required. Wine with insufficient acid, curiously, has a medicinal taste, and does not keep. With too much acid, wine tastes 'sharp' and is slow to make.

Natural acids Cold tea (black) can be used instead of tannin, and natural orange juice and lemon juice are often used in country wines to provide citric acid along with their own citrus fruit flavors. Using dried vine fruits supplies natural grape acids as well as natural sweetness.

Campden tablets

While a must is open to the air there is always the risk of its being affected by transient wild yeasts and bacteria, which can spoil the wine. Campden tablets are an all-purpose sterilizer and stabilizer which prevent spoilage from these agents and kill off wild yeasts already present on your fruit, vegetables, or flowers, so that you can introduce a cultured wine yeast. Because they inhibit the activity of yeast when fresh, 24 hours must elapse before the cultured yeast is added. They may be used in steeping, and at the bottling stage they ensure against contamination and re-fermentation in the bottle. One tablet – the equivalent of just one tenth of a teaspoonful – treats 4.5 liters (1 gallon).

Consisting mainly of potassium or sodium metabisulfite, often incorrectly referred to as metabisulfate, the tablets release sulfur dioxide, explaining why wines have traces of sulfites. However, the sulfur compounds die away as they encounter the aldehydes (alcohol) in wine and any chlorine in the water, so that their presence is negligible in the finished wine. Though Campden tablets are a modern invention, they are widely used in traditional wines now, as a measure against bacterial spoilage, which can occur in even the most hygienically made wines.

What's in a name? Campden tablets get their name from the Cotswolds town of Chipping Campden in Gloucestershire, where they were developed in the 1920s by the Fruit and Vegetable Preserving Research Station. Originally in powder form, to be used in Campden solution, the tablet form was developed by Boots the chemist.

Using Campden tablets Particularly where boiling water is not used, or where ingredients are liable to degrade from oxidation or to become contaminated by long steeping, a Campden tablet can be added in Step 1 to prevent things going wrong. If sterilized bottles are used before they dry in Step 9, Campden tablets are rarely necessary for bottling. Crush one tablet in a saucer using the back of a spoon and add to the ingredients or the finished wine.

Sterilizer (sterilizing solution, sanitizing solution)

Sterilizing solution (this is usually sodium metabisulfite supplied in powder form and made into a solution following the supplier's instructions) must be used to ensure that all winemaking equipment is pristine. Usually this will mean soaking equipment for up to 30 minutes. It is important to make sure that every surface is sterilized. A little sterilizing solution is also used to fill the reservoir in the airlock, and should be replaced after six weeks, if fermenting is still continuing.

Straining

If you use a large straining bag in the fermenting bin in Step 1, all you will need to do is extract it for Step 3 and squeeze it or allow it to drip to extract all the liquid. Otherwise, use a jug and lined straining funnel in Step 3, or pour the contents of the bin through a jumbo straining sieve and into a second container before ladling or siphoning the liquid into the demijohn.

Siphoning/racking

Stand a scrupulously clean second demijohn in the sink and lift the jar that contains the wine onto a safely raised area on the draining board (standing on an upturned bowl, for example). Otherwise, improvise by putting the second demijohn in a large plastic bowl that will catch the splashes and overflow, and stand it on a chair or stool with the wine jar standing on a table. Practice first, with empty containers, to find a way that enables you to have the full jar positioned above the empty one, bearing in mind that when you have transferred the wine to the new demijohn you will have to pick it up. The base of the jar that is full needs to be slightly higher than the top of the empty one. Always move the jar with care so as to disturb the sediment as little as possible.

When racking, gently twist out the bung and airlock, dip one end of your sterilized tubing into the full jar, keeping it away from the lees, and suck the other end until the wine starts to travel down the tube. Take the tube out of your mouth, cover the end with a finger or thumb, and guide it into position over the mouth of the second jar via a funnel. Let go and the wine will run into the jar. For total hygiene, it is possible to use a purpose-made device to get the wine flowing, so that your mouth is not in contact with the tube. Fit an airlock into the new jar and transfer it back into position.

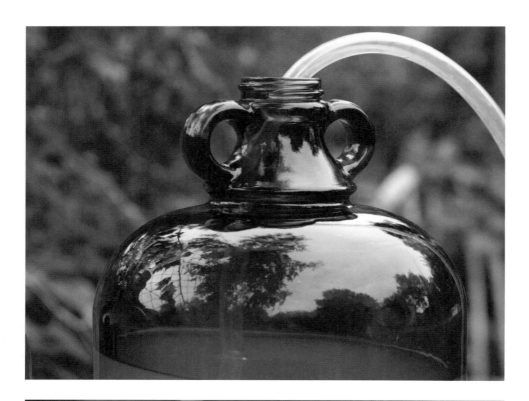

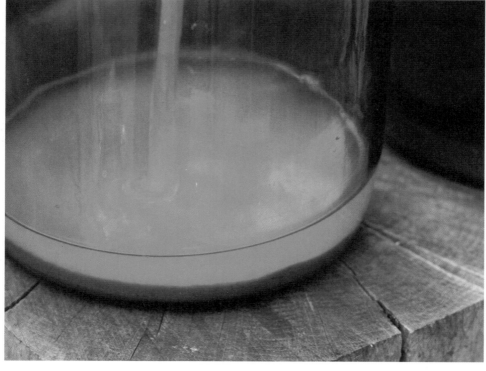

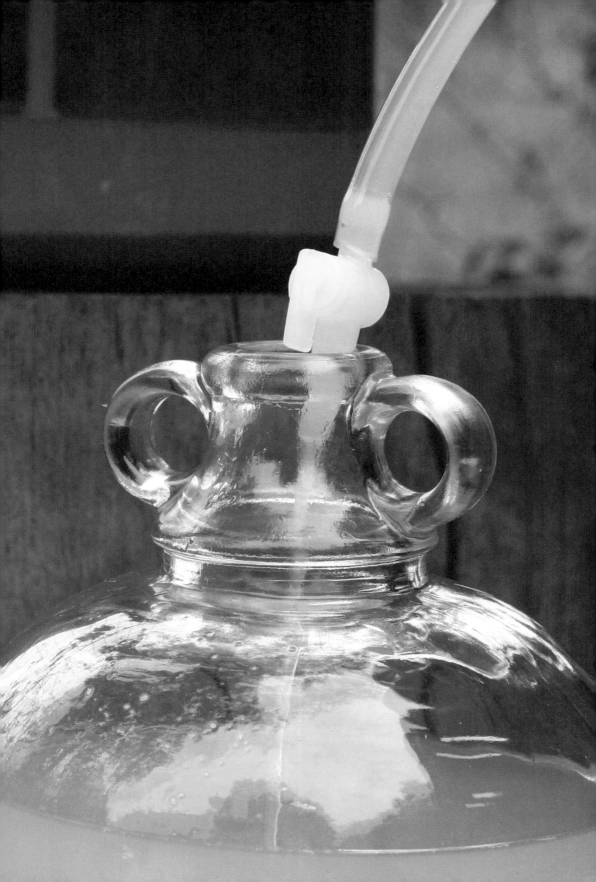

Racking will usually need to be carried out twice, once after about a week and then again as the wine clears and fermentation slows down, but it should be done whenever a thick sediment has formed. Leaving the liquid too long on the lees can cause off-flavors in the wine and hinder its clarification.

Waste not, want not If you have a garden, use the lees as fertilizer.

Topping up You will probably find that after racking there is less liquid in the second jar than there was in the first. You can top up with cool sugar syrup (see page 34) or with any surplus must that you have been saving.

Fining/finings

Fining clarifies the finished wine and in commercial wines is also used to reduce the tannin content if this is too high. It is generally not essential for country wines, especially if you have ended up with a clear bright wine when fermentation is complete. Sometimes, however, wine remains clouded with very fine particles after fermentation, either because of extremely starchy ingredients or because it was strained initially through an insufficiently fine strainer. Traditionally this was remedied by floating baked eggshells in the wine, but it is simpler to use purpose-made finings, which will clear the wine quite rapidly if used according to the manufacturer's instructions. A much-used product is Vin Clear.

Fine point Using finings does present a slight problem for vegetarians, since many fining ingredients are based on animal products. Gelatin is a traditional ingredient (its use leaves a slight sediment which then has to be filtered out before bottling). Other sources of fining agents are bull's blood, animal bone, and isinglass, from sturgeon bladder. Finings based on casein and lysozyme from milk, or albumin from eggs, are obtainable. Filtering to clarify the wine can be done with paper filters if needed.

Potassium sorbate/stabilizer

This is a safe but effective antioxidant that is often used in conjunction with Campden tablets to stabilize and protect the color of the finished wine, particularly with wines that tend to go off color during storage. This use also helps prevent further unwanted fermentation occurring in the bottles. Potassium sorbate can also be used to prevent oxidation during steeping and open fermentation.

Vitamin C (ascorbic acid)

This is a natural antioxidant and can be used at the bottling stage to maintain the delicate color of some wines. It also safeguards the nutritional constituents of fruits and vegetables. Vitamin C can be obtained in powder or tablet form.

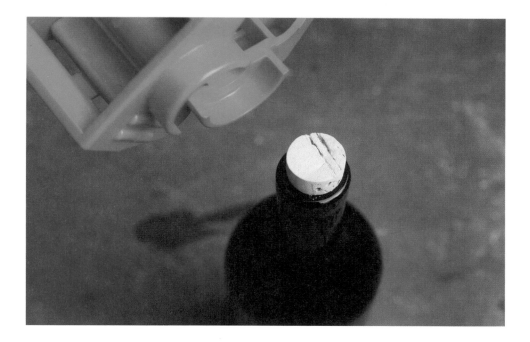

Bottling

Aerating the wine before bottling does it good, and helps to release any trapped carbon dioxide. One technique for bottling is to transfer the cleared wine to an open container (sterilized first) and from there ladle it into bottles using a jug and funnel. The more professional way is to siphon (see page 39) the finished wine into the sterilized bottles. Either way, it is advisable to stand the bottles in a large plastic bowl or at least on a layer of newspaper, as there will be drips and splashes. Cork securely, using sterilized corks. After corking, wipe clean the outside of the bottles with a clean cloth wrung out in sterilizing solution.

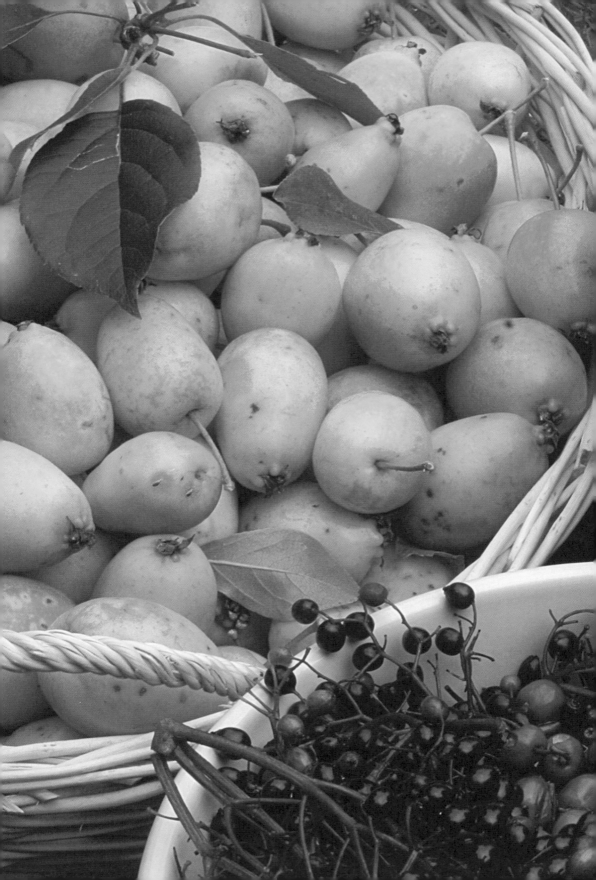

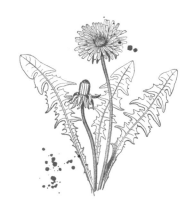

FORAGING

Many of the ingredients for the wines in this book will be found in the wild, though others will be purchased, grown, or given away.

First catch your crop

Whether you use flowers, fruits, or vegetables, and whether they are wild or cultivated, there are a few golden rules.

* Be sure of what you are picking.

* Be sure that you have a right to pick it.

* Pick only what you need and know you are going to use.

* Don't damage the plant.

* Don't damage the surroundings in getting access to the plant.

* Don't use plants growing close to roads or near to fields that have recently been treated with pesticide or herbicide.

* Pick at the stage of maturity unless the recipe specifies differently. For example, under-ripe fruit will be too sour and not juicy enough, over-ripe fruit will have lost its flavor and may have started to be contaminated by natural molds which affect the flavor of the wine.

* When using windfalls, check the fruits carefully before using them, and cut away any bruised or damaged parts. Reject fruits that are under- or over-ripe.

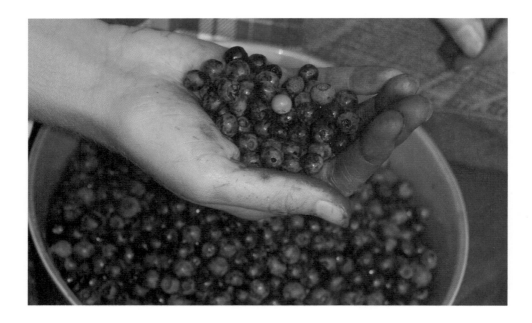

Take containers with you on your country walks. For blackberries a stout walking stick will come in handy to pull down the canes as well as a rigid container such as a plastic ice-cream box or cooking fat box, well washed but dry and with a lid. A country basket is a charming accessory for wild fruit gathering, and will ensure that the fruit doesn't get squashed, but make sure that it is big enough for the amount you need so that there will be no spills. Strong plastic bags are acceptable as long as you don't leave your bounty in them to stew and as long as you make sure that the content doesn't get squashed on the way home. Large, strong paper bags, tucked inside a plastic bag are better. Fairly rigid canvas bags with a gusset so that they stand up on their own, are better still. And some canny gatherers save time and trouble by picking straight into a measuring bin, so they know just how much they have picked.

Some wild plants have legal protection, and it is illegal to dig up wild plants. Many wild plants that were once common are now endangered or rare. You will do no harm if you stick to the plants and advice in these recipes, as long as you harvest carefully, gathering a little from a number of plants, resisting when plants are rare in the local area, and using a knife or scissors for cutting through stems or removing leaves.

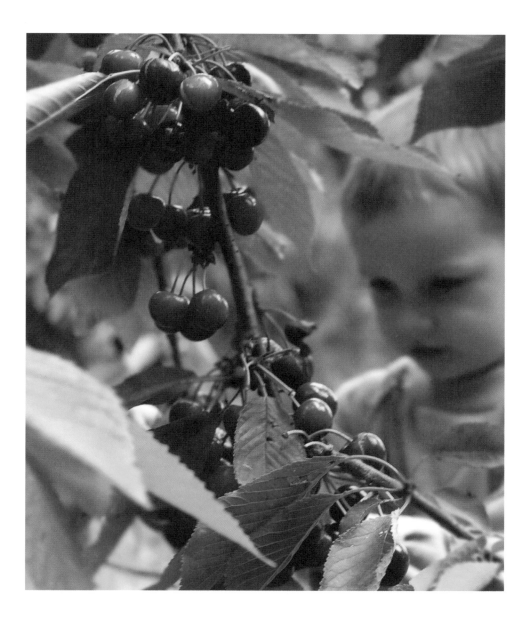

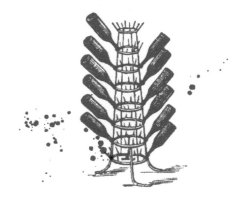

TROUBLESHOOTING

This part of the book lists things that might go wrong in making wild wine or country wine, and explains their possible causes. Some of these may sound awful – but they are not a reason to be put off. Sometimes the problems can be remedied after the event, and usually they can be prevented with a bit of forward preparation. So, if you read the problem section before you start to make your wine, you will be on the lookout and – we hope – be able to avoid the problem before you encounter it.

Fermentation is sluggish or stops (called 'sticking')

The most likely cause is the temperature (see below). Too much heat slows down fermentation and can even kill the yeast, but not enough heat slows down or inactivates most yeasts. Different yeasts may require different temperatures, so check the sachet instructions for the yeast you are using.

Open fermentation should not cause this problem unless you forgot to put in the yeast – as long as you allowed 24 hours to elapse between using a Campden tablet and adding the yeast, and as long as the room is warm enough and with no drafts. The temperature should be at a constant 18–24°C (65–75°F). A very high temperature (over 35°C/95°F) will kill the yeast completely, which is why boiled ingredients must be allowed to cool before yeast is added. A high temperature (going over 27°C/80°F) can adversely affect the taste.

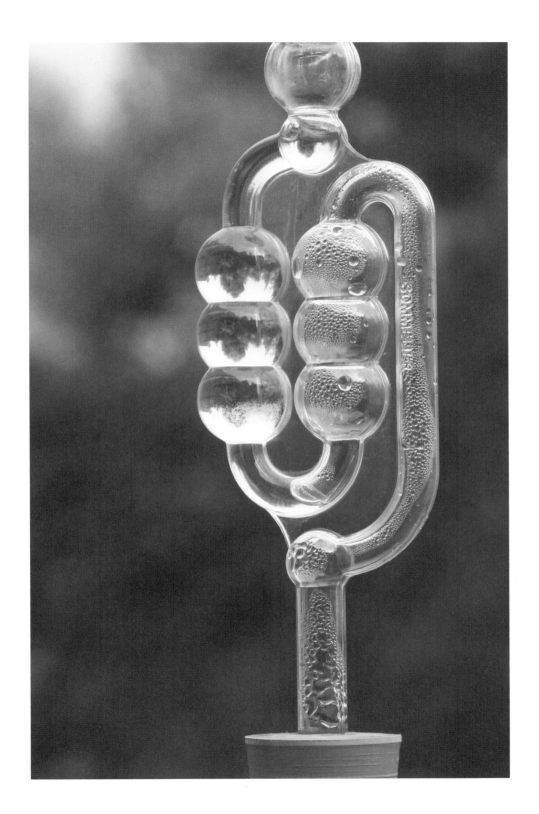

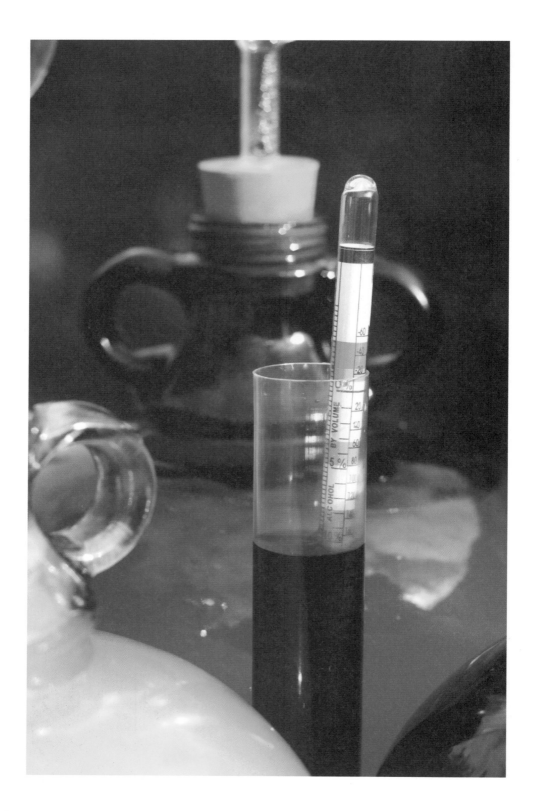

If you think the yeast may have been affected by a Campden tablet, give the mix three good stirs, once an hour. If nothing happens within five hours, make up some more yeast and add it to the container.

Closed fermentation The jar should be adequately warm, but high temperatures discourage yeast activity. The activity of closed fermentation adds about 5°C (10°F) to the temperature inside the jar, so a lower surrounding temperature is needed than in open fermentation, and this should be constant, at about 16°C (60°F).

Other possible causes of sticking

Insufficient nutrient As long as you have used a yeast and nutrient combined, this should not occur.

The sugar has been used up If fermentation has stopped too soon, try drawing off a little of the must and adding a little sugar. Keep it warm for up to four hours. If there is a reaction, you can add more sugar to the jar – at worst you will have a sweeter wine. Add extra sugar a spoonful at a time, not in one go.

The yeast has failed If the above remedies have no effect, make up another batch of yeast (see page 35).

Low acid This can be the case with flower and vegetable wines and with certain fruits. Use the amount of acid blend or citrus fruit juice specified in the recipe.

Trapped gas Try removing the bung and replacing it with cotton wool for a day or two. Also check that you have not over-filled the airlock reservoir.

Fermentation is finished Move the jar to a warmer place for a couple of days to check this. If there is no more bubbling, it is time to bottle the wine.

Wine does not clear during fermenting

Some wines take a long time to clear, and require frequent racking. Take care when racking not to transfer any of the sediment with the wine.

Finished wine is cloudy

All wines should clear within nine months to a year. Moving the jar to a cooler place when fermentation stops should lead to the wine's clearing in about a month. Failing this, use finings (see page 42).

Wine has a haze

This is different from failing to clear. The haze will be white, light purple, or brownish, and is a sign of contamination, usually caused by using metal equipment (other than stainless steel or enamel-ware). It is best to throw away the wine and learn the lesson.

Wine appears hazed

Check the must carefully to make sure that this really is a haze. Powdery flecks forming in the wine and gathering on the surface are not a haze but a sign of bacterial contamination known as 'flowers in the wine'. This can be remedied if spotted early by filtering the wine into a clean demijohn through a very fine filter and adding two crushed Campden tablets. Add a fresh batch of yeast after 24 hours and continue with fermentation.

An 'oil slick' in the wine

This is what is known as 'ropey' wine and can be caused by a suspension of sugar or by the presence of lactic acid. It is harmless but unsightly. Treat as for flowers in the wine (see above).

An off flavor

This can be caused by standing the wine for too long on the lees. Frequent racking will prevent it, but there is no treatment after the event.

Medicinal taste

This is often due to too little acid in the ingredients. It cannot be remedied in the finished wine. Always use the amount of acid specified in the ingredients. Wine with too little acid also fails to keep.

'Sharp' taste

With too much acid, wine tastes 'sharp' and is slow to make. If your wine took a long time in the making, this will probably be the cause and the result.

Vinegar taste

Your wine is vinegar! It is vital to keep away tiny flies known as vinegar flies, which appear from nowhere at the slightest hint of fermentation. This is why a cover is used even during open fermentation. The flies can also be attracted during closed fermentation, and the airlock must be kept firmly in place, and filled with sterilizing solution, which is replaced every five or six weeks.

Bottles explode or corks pop out in storage

This happens if fermentation starts up in the bottle, either because you bottled before fermentation was complete or, in sweet wine, because the wine was not stabilized. The solution is to open any bottles that have not yet exploded and re-ferment in a demijohn.

In sparkling wines, where fermentation in the bottles is what makes the sparkle, it can be due to the bottles not being of Champagne quality or to the corks not being properly secured. It may be possible to rescue some of the wine and rebottle it.

Musty smell when the wine is opened

Reusing old corks or insufficiently sterilizing the corks can cause the wine to be musty ('corked'). Prevent this by using only new and well-sterilized corks and don't store the wine in a damp environment. It is sometimes possible to save the remaining wine by removing the corks, cleaning the bottle necks with a sterilizing solution-soaked cloth and recorking with properly prepared corks.

Yeasty-tasting wine

This can be caused by using non-wine yeast, insufficient racking, or too short a storage period.

Oxidation

A 'browning' of the wine and a slightly bitter taste. These are caused by using over-ripe fruit or insufficient acid, and failure to stabilize oxidation-prone wines.

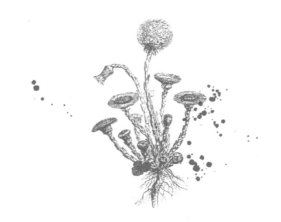

FLOWER WINES

Flowers lend the most delicate flavors to wild wines, though they normally lack acids, sugars, and juices. Generally, the flavors are extracted by making an infusion with boiling water or by steeping the flowers in cold water for a longer period. The infusion is then mixed with vital acids and other ingredients to balance the taste, yeast and sugar are added, and possibly vine fruit to give the wine some body. Usually, but not always, only the flowers themselves are used, with as little of the stalk and green part of the plant as possible, but occasionally the whole stems are used in the infusion to make a more herbal wine. A small quantity of dried flowers can be used instead of fresh when the fresh ones cannot be found, and wild flower seeds and plant plugs are available from several specialist suppliers for anyone who would like to grow them in the garden or on a balcony. These wines are often ready to drink quite quickly and don't need a long storing time.

Agrimony
Agrimonia eupatoria
also known as Sticklewort, Cockleburr
A native of the British Isles and northern Europe, Agrimony is a wayside plant with spikes of starry yellow flowers growing singly up a tall and gently twisting stem. The flowers are larger towards the base of the hairy stems, decreasing upward in size, with smaller flowers clustered closely at the top.

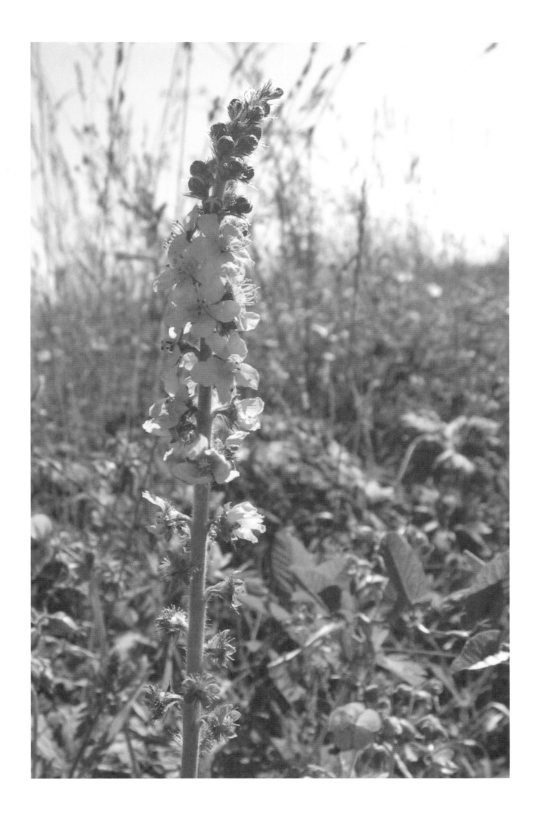

The hairy leaves grow widely separated up the flower stems. Each has seven or nine leaflets arranged as pairs topped with a single leaflet, and with tiny leaflets separating them.

The flowering stems, which can be branching, are generally about 60 cm (2 ft) high, but are sometimes shorter, and in some parts of the world can grow to twice this height. The five-petalled flowers ripen into little burrs that will cling to the clothing of passers-by. The plant is a perennial with a short, woody, creeping rootstock, reddish in color.

The whole plant is lightly but pleasantly scented, and has long been used in folk medicine and herbalism as a remedy for 'liverishness.'

You'll find it flowering in mid- to late summer, in field and woodland edges, in waste places, and by roadsides. Agrimony grows wild in North America and can be found almost worldwide. Pick the flowers on a dry, sunny day.

Sweet Agrimony Wine

The lemons and orange in this recipe supply acidity and extra flavor, while raisins give a fruity roundness. As an astringent herb, Agrimony is rich in tannin, so no additional tannin is required.

You will need
* 1 medium-sized bunch of Agrimony
* 2 lemons, pared and squeezed
* 1 orange, pared and squeezed
* 1 Campden tablet, crushed
* 4.5 liters (1 gallon) water
* yeast and nutrient
* 1.3 kg (3 lb) sugar
* 225 g (8 oz) raisins, chopped

Method

1   Place the flower spikes and leaves in a large container. Add the pared zest and the crushed Campden tablet.

2   Boil the water and pour it over the flower mix. Cover and leave to steep for two days, stirring twice daily. Activate the yeast toward the end of this time (see page 35).

3   Put the sugar into the fermenting bin and strain the flower infusion over it, stirring until the sugar is completely dissolved.

4   Add the chopped raisins, lemon and orange juice, and activated yeast.

5   Cover and leave to ferment vigorously for five days, stirring twice daily and pressing down the cap that rises to the surface.

6   Strain the liquid into a demijohn, fit the airlock, and carry on with closed fermentation, racking as the sediment forms.

7   When fermentation is complete and the wine is clear, bottle, cork, and label. Store in a cool place for four months.

Note

*   You can use one 75 g (2½ oz) packet of dried Agrimony flowers instead of fresh flowers for this wine.

Clover
Trifolium pratense (**Red Clover**)
Trifolium repens (**White Clover**)
also known as Purple Clover and White Clover

These are the well-known Common Clovers of fields and grasslands, loved by bees for their sweet nectar. The name *trifolium* means three leaves or leaflets, and hunt as you may you will not find a four-leaved clover. The honey-scented flowers, which form dense, rounded heads, bloom from very early summer until the autumn and can be used to make a fragrant country wine.

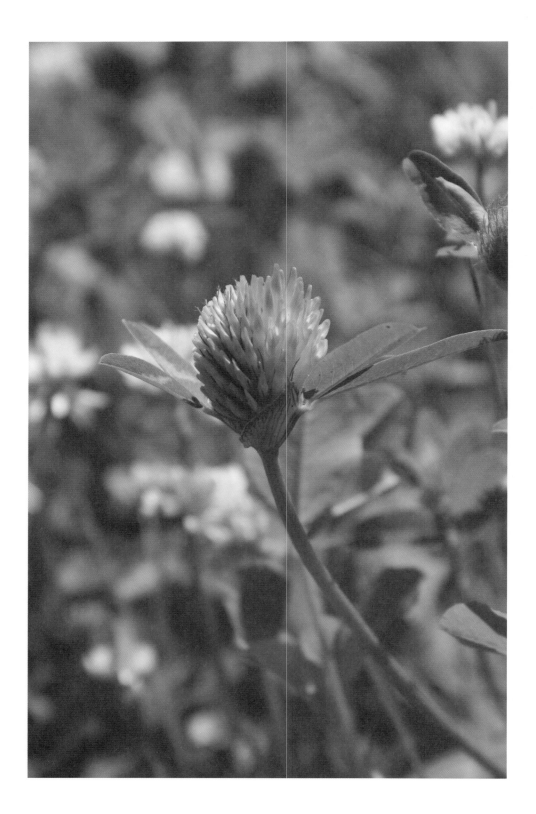

Red Clover flowers on stems 25 cm (10 in) or more high and its flowers are more purple or deep pink than red, hence its common name of Purple Clover. White Clover has a creeping habit and its flower stalks are often only 10 cm (4 in) high. It withstands low mowing and survives in garden lawns however severely they are cut. Both Clovers reach a greater height in uncut grass.

You'll find it in hay-meadows and open areas of grass- and pastureland, especially in fertile, light, or sandy soils. Clovers are also cultivated as a crop to nourish the soil and can be grown in the garden when space allows.

Work for the bees Darwin noted that Red Clover could not exist without 'humble-bees', because, while many other insects are pollinators, only the bees' tongues are long enough to fertilize the Clover flowers as they feed on the nectar.

Clover Wine

Use the flower heads only for this light and summery wine, separated from the stems and without any leaves. Measure them by volume, pressed down lightly in a marked container. Dried flowers can also be used.

You will need
* 2.3–3 liters (4–6 pints) Clover flowers
* 1 Campden tablet, crushed
* 4.5 liters (1 gallon) water
* yeast and nutrient (see note on page 60)
* 1.3 kg (3 lb) sugar
* 225 g (8 oz) sultanas, chopped
* 2.5 ml (½ teaspoon) grape tannin
* 2 lemons, pared and squeezed
* 2 oranges, pared and squeezed

Method

1 Measure the flowers into a fermenting bin and mix in the crushed Campden tablet. Bring the water to a boil and pour it over the flowers. Cover and leave to infuse.

2 After about 24 hours, activate the yeast (see page 35). Pour the sugar into the bin and stir well to dissolve it, then add the chopped sultanas and grape tannin and stir in the zest and juice of the lemons and oranges.

3 When the yeast is working, add it to the bin, cover, and leave to ferment in a warm place for five days, stirring twice daily and pressing down the cap.

4 Strain the liquid into a demijohn, fit the airlock and leave to ferment. Rack as the sediment forms.

5 When fermentation is complete and the wine is clear, bottle, cork, and label. Store in a cool place for four months.

Notes

* A Champagne yeast works well with this delicately pink-hued wine.
* You can use 100 g (4 oz) dried flowers instead of fresh ones in Step 1.

Coltsfoot

Tussilago farfara

also known as Clerk of the Weather, Coughwort, Foal's-foot

In earlier times Coltsfoot was a favorite harbinger of spring, as the plant is so quick to respond to the departure of winter that it flowers before its leaves appear. Its old name of Clerk of the Weather comes from this haste to burst into action once the winter is truly at an end – and the plant seldom makes a mistake.

Very widely found in the British Isles and Europe, and in most parts of North America, Coltsfoot has daisy-like flowers with a mass of narrow, clear yellow petals radiating from a sunny yellow disc, which itself has stubby little petals. The sturdy, low-growing stems – some 15 cm (6 in) high – are flesh-pink to pale buff, with woolly scales, each stem bearing one flower. The stems grow in clusters and the roughly heart-shaped leaves (resembling the footprints of a young colt) start to surface among them as the flowers turn into downy seedheads.

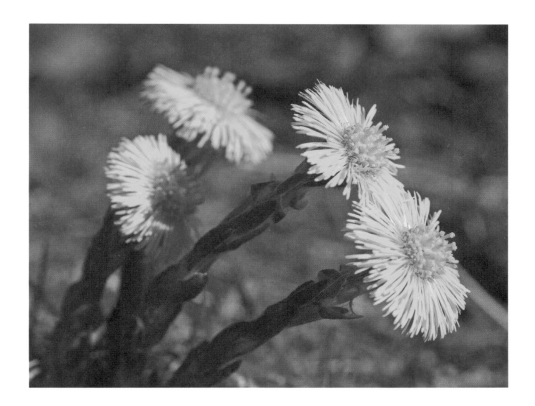

Historically, this plant was much used in the treatment of coughs, as its name tells us (cough = *tussis* in Latin). Country people had great faith in its curative powers, and Coltsfoot wine was a staunch household favorite.

You'll find it growing in a sunny spot in waste places, wet or dry, particularly in loamy or shingly soils and on limestone; also on banks and dunes. It can be hard to find, but where it does grow it forms cheerful colonies. Use scissors to cut the flowers you need.

Caution There has recently been some evidence that large amounts of Coltsfoot taken over a long period can be harmful to health. It is therefore suggested that Coltsfoot wine should be drunk in small quantities.

Environment concern Once a very common plant of early spring, Coltsfoot seems to be much rarer today. Therefore you should only gather the plant if you find it growing in extensive colonies. Instead, try growing it from seed or plug plants in a patch in the garden, or use the dried herb.

Coltsfoot Wine

The Demerara sugar in this recipe complements the Coltsfoot flavor. For a real country touch, try using a small cup of cold tea instead of tannin. Remove the flowers from the stems and measure them in a container, pressed down lightly.

You will need
* 2.3 liters (4 pints) Coltsfoot flowers (or 100 g/4 oz dried flowers)
* 1 Campden tablet, crushed
* 4.5 liters (1 gallon) water
* yeast and nutrient
* 2 oranges, pared and squeezed
* 2 lemons, pared and squeezed
* 225 g (8 oz) chopped raisins
* 1.3 kg (3 lb) Demerara sugar
* 2.5 ml (½ teaspoon) grape tannin
* 1 small cup cold tea (optional, see Method)

Method
1   Place the flowers in a large container, add the crushed Campden tablet, and bring the water to a boil. Pour the boiling water over the flowers, cover, and leave to steep for three days, stirring twice daily.
2   Activate the yeast toward the end of this time (see page 35).
3   Put the zest and juices of the oranges and lemons into a fermenting bin with the raisins, add the sugar, and strain the infused Coltsfoot liquid onto the mixture. Stir well to make sure that the sugar is dissolved.
4   Add the tannin (or tea) and activated yeast. Cover and leave in a warm place to ferment for up to a week. Continue to stir twice daily, and press down the cap that rises to the surface during this time.
5   Strain the must into a demijohn, fit the airlock, and leave to continue fermenting. Rack the wine once or twice as it clears.
6   Bottle, cork, and label when fermentation is complete and the wine is clear. Store for at least one year before tasting this wine.

Dandelion

Taraxacum officinale

also known as Clocks and Watches, Priest's Crown, Wet the Bed

Dandelions may be a pain in the lawn, but a field of golden yellow Dandelions is a fine sight in mid-spring. The flowers attract the early bees and the Dandelion seedheads make 'cuckoo clocks' by which country children still tell the time as the downy seeds fly off into the air when the children blow on them. The hollow stems contain a white, milky, rubbery substance which stains the hands brown and was used as a cure for warts, and the flowers have a slightly herbal scent all of their own which gives a distinctive flavor to Dandelion wine.

The flowering stems have a height of 10 cm (4 in) or more, and the flowers grow singly on the stems, surrounded at the base by bunches of dark green leaves with very jagged edges and a pronounced central rib. The plant has a strong, woody tap root, which (as gardeners know) drives itself deep into the ground, and which exudes a milky sap when cut. Flowers, leaves, and roots are all very beneficial to health, and have been used as a general springtime tonic. All parts of the plant taste bitter: the leaves can be eaten in salads and the root is roasted and ground to make a healthy substitute for coffee. The flowers themselves are best reserved for wine.

You'll find it in great profusion in grassy fields and meadows, waysides, waste places, and garden lawns, especially in the sun.

Recognition The hollow milky stems should help to identify Dandelions. The flowers are a dense mass of petals of a bright golden yellow, and the outer ones are reddish-brown on the back.

Dandelion Wine

Dandelion Wine has a long pedigree and is said to be a tonic. Tasting slightly of sherry, it is a wine to be sipped. If you have the patience to pull the petals from the flower heads after measuring the volume required, you will be rewarded with a more refined wine.

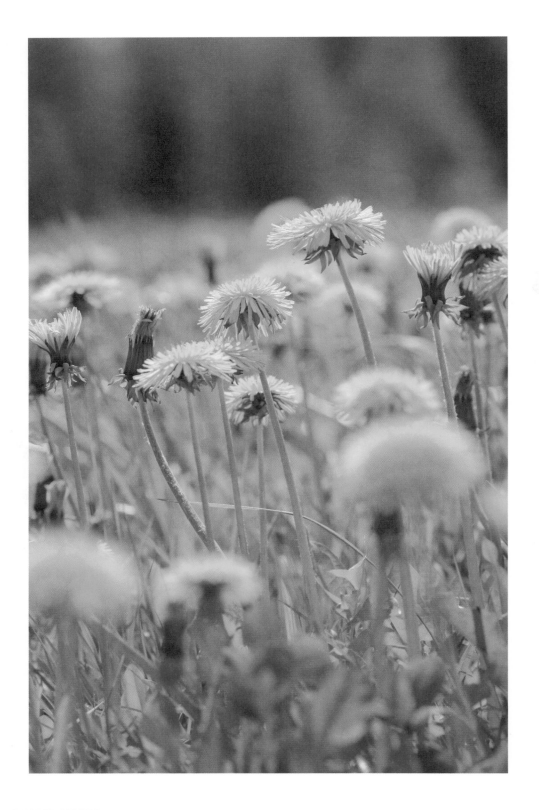

You will need

* 4.5 liters (1 gallon) Dandelion flowers, loosely packed
* 1 Campden tablet, crushed
* 4.5 liters (1 gallon) water
* 1.6 kg (3½ lb) sugar
* small piece of ginger root, sliced
* 1 orange, pared and squeezed
* 1 lemon, pared and squeezed
* 2.5 ml (½ teaspoon) grape tannin
* yeast and nutrient

Optional extras (see note below)

* 225 g (8 oz) sultanas, chopped
* 1 small cup cold tea

Method

1   Place the flowers and crushed Campden tablet in a container and pour 4.5 liters (1 gallon) of boiling water over them.
2   Stir well, cover, and leave to steep for two days, stirring once or twice daily.
3   Strain about one third of the liquor into a pan and bring it to a boil, boil for 10 minutes, then put the sugar into a fermenting bin and pour the hot infusion over it.
4   Stir until the sugar has dissolved and add the sliced ginger root, the juice and zest of the orange and lemon, and the tannin. Strain and boil the remaining liquor in convenient quantities and pour into the bin.
5   When the liquid has cooled to blood heat (21–24°C/70–75°F), sprinkle in the yeast and nutrient.
6   Cover and leave for about five days in a warm place, stirring twice daily.
7   When open fermentation has calmed down, strain the liquid into a demijohn and fit the airlock. Ferment, racking as the sediment forms.
8   When fermentation is complete and the wine is clear, bottle, cork, and label. Store for a year before using.

Note

* This wine was once so popular that there are many versions. Raisins or sultanas can be added with the sugar and cold tea can be used instead of tannin.

Elderflower
Sambucus nigra
also known as Black Elder, Bore or Bour Tree, European Elder
The Elder tree is a native of most parts of Europe and a close relation, known as Canadian Elder, is found in North America. In late spring and early summer, both bear saucers of foaming, lacy flowers which can be used for wines, cordial, and Elderflower 'Champagne.' In early autumn the dark purple fruits will give a second harvest for wine and syrup (see page 106 for details).

Elders grow in many shapes and sizes, from shrubby bushes to small or larger trees, up to 9 m (30 ft) in height, but very often lower. The leaves consist of two to four pairs of leaflets topped with a single leaflet and they have a distinctive bitter scent when crushed. The flowers likewise have a most distinctive fragrance, sweet but sharp, and scenting the surrounding air. The bark is rough and cork-like, especially on older trees, and the branches used to be hollowed out to make musical instruments.

The creamy white flowers are tiny individually, but grow by the dozen on little branching stalks, forming flat heads of blossom up to 20 cm (8 in) across. The newly opened flowers growing in full sun have the most pleasing perfume and are best for wine.

You'll find it in hedges and woodland and in waste ground, especially in damp places near streams, ponds, and ditches.

Elderflower Wine
Slow to finish fermenting but quick to mature, this is a wine that really has all the fragrance of the flowers. Elderflowers can also easily and quickly be made into a light and delicately flavored sparkling 'wine' that is perfect for special occasions.

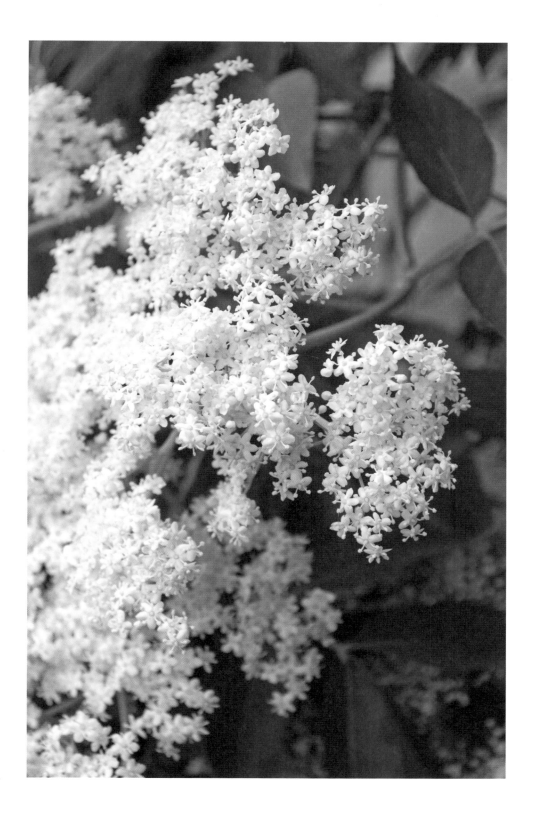

You will need

* 1.2–1.7 liters (2–3 pints) by volume of Elder blossoms
* 1.3 kg (3 lb) sugar
* 225 g (8 oz) sultanas, chopped
* 2 lemons, squeezed
* 2.5 ml (½ teaspoon) grape tannin
* 4.5 liters (1 gallon) water
* Champagne yeast or Hock yeast (all-purpose yeast may also be used)

Method

1   Prepare the flowers by using scissors to remove the florets from the stems, leaving as little of the stem as possible. This should produce about 600 ml (1 pint) of flowers, when pressed down.

2   Put the flowers, sugar, sultanas, lemon juice, tannin, and water into the fermenting bin. Stir, cover, and leave for 24 hours to infuse.

3   Activate the yeast (see page 35) and add it to the infusion. Cover, transfer to a warm place, and allow the yeast to ferment for six or seven days, stirring twice daily.

4   Strain into a demijohn, fit the airlock, and leave to ferment, racking as the sediment forms. Fermentation may take several months.

5   When bubbling has ceased, move the jar to a slightly warmer place for a day or two to make quite sure that the yeast is not still active. Then rack again, bottle, cork, and label. Store for four months before drinking.

Elderflower 'Champagne'

This sparkling drink is ready for use in two weeks, but tastes even better after being stored in a cool place for six months. No yeast is required.

You will need

* 6 large Elderflower heads
* 4.5 liters (1 gallon) cold water
* 560 g (1¼ lb) sugar
* 30 ml (2 tablespoons) white wine vinegar
* 1 lemon, finely pared and squeezed

Method

1 Snip the flowers from the stalks and put them in a large deep jar.
2 Pour on the water and add the sugar, wine vinegar, and lemon zest and juice.
3 Stir thoroughly to dissolve the sugar.
4 Cover the jar and leave it to stand in a cool place for 24 hours.
5 Strain off the liquid and bottle it straight away in strong, screw-cap bottles. The 'wine' will soon start to fizz, so check the bottles every few days and release any excess pressure by gently unscrewing the caps. Drink before the year is up.

Note

* Glass sparkling-mineral-water bottles are the kind to use.

Gorse

Ulex europaeus

also known as Furze, Furzes, Prickly Broom or Prickley Broome, Whins

Gorse is a member of the Pea family, often confused with Broom. Many old recipes for 'Broom Wine' were almost certainly intended for Gorse flowers. While Broom is smooth of stem and relatively graceful, Gorse makes a thorny, prickly bush, growing to 3 m (10 ft) high, and forming dense thickets. These act as a buffer to the wind in open spaces and provide shelter for wildlife and grazing animals.

The dark green stems are furrowed and the plant has spines instead of leaves. The golden yellow flowers have a scent of warm coconut, and the pods dry and crack open on a sunny day to release the seeds. Native to western Europe and very common throughout that region, Gorse is in flower almost all year but prolifically so from mid-spring to mid-summer.

You'll find it growing in heaths, commons, moors, and scrubland, and on the top of chalk downs. Gorse bushes are distinguished to the forager by their sharp spines, which make picking the scented yellow flowers an adventure.

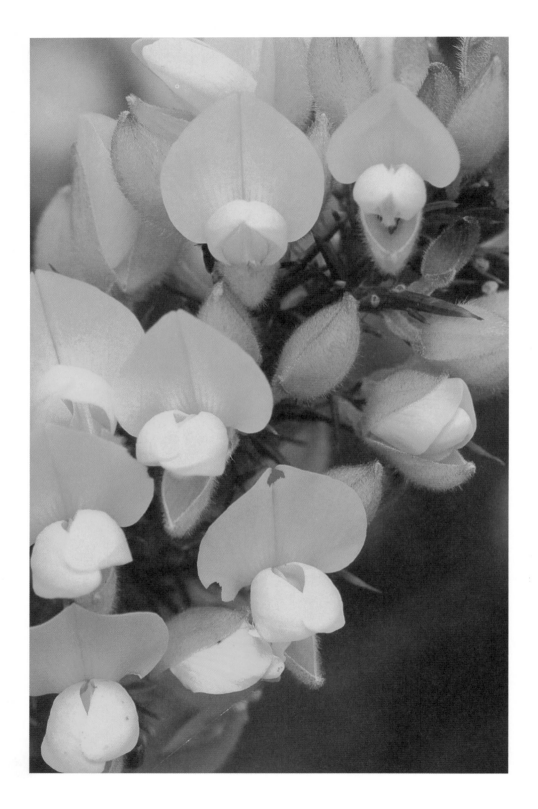

Gorse Wine

This makes a fairly sweet wine with a pale yellow hue, which preserves the subtle scent of the flowers and repays all the effort of picking and preparing them. Oranges seem to suit the flavor better than lemons but lemons could be used.

You will need

* 2.3 liters (4 pints) Gorse flowers, pressed down
* 1 Campden tablet, crushed
* 4.5 liters (1 gallon) boiling water
* 225 g (8 oz) sultanas, minced
* 3 oranges, thinly pared and squeezed
* 2.5 ml (½ teaspoon) grape tannin or 175 ml (6 fl oz) strong tea
* 1.3 kg (3 lb) sugar
* yeast and nutrient

Method

1   Put the Gorse flowers with the crushed Campden tablet into a large container, pour on the boiling water, cover, and leave to infuse for two days, stirring once or twice a day.
2   Strain the liquid into a fermenting bin into which you have put the sultanas, fruit zest and juice, tannin or tea, and sugar.
3   Stir well to make sure that the sugar is completely dissolved and activate the yeast (see page 35).
4   When the yeast is bubbling, add it to the container, cover, and leave to ferment in a warm place for a week, stirring daily and pushing down the sultanas.
5   Transfer to a demijohn and fit the airlock. Leave to ferment in a warm place, racking the wine from the sediment as it clears.
6   When fermentation has stopped and the wine is completely clear, carefully strain into a container and cork tightly. Leave to mature for several months, then bottle, cork, and label. Store for one year before opening.

Hawthorn Blossom

Crataegus monogyna

also known as Common Hawthorn, English Hawthorn, May Blossom, Whitethorn

Heavily scented, Hawthorn or May Blossom is redolent of late spring and the promise of summer. Some people find the scent unpleasant and it is true that it is close to being overpowering. It is probably for this reason that May is said to be unlucky if brought indoors, where its perfume can hang in a room – but carried by the air on a day of blue skies and breezes it surely cannot fail to stir the spirits.

The Hawthorn is a native of the British Isles and continental Europe, and as far east as Afghanistan, but can also be found in North America. A bush or small tree up to 6 m (20 ft) high (or more, if left to its own devices) and often planted as hedging, Hawthorn is covered in white or pink-flushed flowers in mid-spring. The flowers are like tiny single roses, with cupped petals and a central boss of stamens, covered with pink pollen as they open, black when the pollen has been taken by the many flying insects it attracts. Small and deeply lobed, the leaves open fresh and light spring green and soon grow dark and almost leathery in texture. When first in bud, they used to be gathered by country children and eaten raw as 'bread and cheese.'

A wonderful wild plant for winemakers, Hawthorn provides both flowers and fruit (see page 115) in plenty.

You'll find it on open farmland, in woodland margins and in field hedges, especially on chalky soils. Pick the flowers when they are young and fresh.

Folk weather lore The more plentiful the May Blossom, the more this is supposed to portend a good summer on the way.

Hawthorn Blossom Wine

also known as May Blossom Wine

Here is a pale, clear wine to remind you of the early days of summer. Whether drinking it will help your love life – or keep away witches – as May Blossom was once supposed to do, is a matter for conjecture.

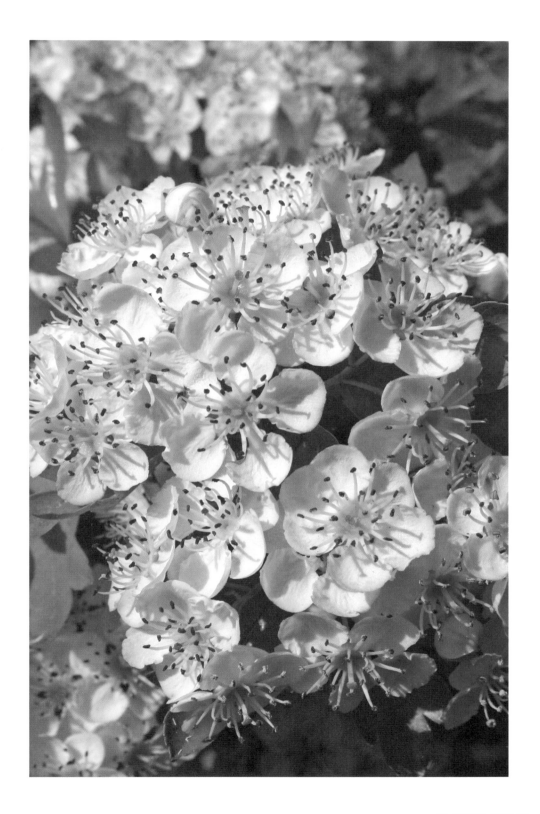

You will need

* 2.3 liters (4 pints) May blossoms
* 1.3 kg (3 lb) sugar
* 5 ml (1 teaspoon) grape tannin
* 1 lemon, thinly pared and squeezed
* 1 orange, thinly pared and squeezed
* 4.5 liters (1 gallon) boiling water
* yeast and nutrient

Method

1 Cut off the flowers from their stems and put them into a fermenting bin. Add the sugar, tannin, and lemon and orange parings, pour on the boiling water, stir well, cover and leave to cool to blood heat (21–24°C/70–75°F).

2 Take a little of the warm infusion in a clean cup or jug and dissolve the yeast into it.

3 Stir the lemon and orange juice into the infusion and add the yeast.

4 Cover and leave to ferment for three days, stirring twice daily and pushing down the cap that forms on the surface.

5 Strain into a demijohn, plug the mouth with clean cotton wool and keep in a warm place for two more days, wiping up any froth that spills over, and replacing the cotton wool if necessary.

6 Fit the airlock after this time, and allow fermentation to continue, racking the wine from the sediment as it clears.

7 When fermentation has ceased and the wine is completely clear, remove to a cool place for two weeks, then bottle, cork, and label. Store for four months before opening.

Marigold

Calendula officinalis

also known as Calendula, Mary Bud, Pot Marigold

Marigold is an aromatic garden plant that may escape into the wild on waste land or at the edge of fields near to gardens. Since at least the Middle Ages it has been cultivated by herbalists for its medicinal properties, and grown in gardens for home remedies and other household uses. The name 'Pot Marigold' comes from the fact that the dried petals were used in winter soups and stews and they were also added to cheeses and butter to improve their color. A native of central and southern Europe, and parts of Asia, it is now grown all over the world.

The flowers of Marigold are brightly colored in shades of orange and yellow, with quilled petals radiating from an open center. Single and double forms are available, and the plants grow best in well-drained soil and an open, sunny position. The grey-green leaves, arranged in spirals on the stems, are sticky to the touch, as are the ridged and branching stems. The plant grows to a height of up to 75 cm (30 in), depending on the variety.

You will not usually find this plant growing in the wild, and it is very easy to grow in a garden or window box. Just sow the seeds in early spring, or in late summer for earlier flowers the following year. Though it is an annual that needs to be grown from scratch each year, the plant soon self-seeds in open ground. The common, single, orange kind is best for household use, including winemaking.

Mistaken identity The garden Marigold (*Calendula*) is a different plant from the more showy French Marigold and African Marigold (both *Tagetes* varieties), which come from Mexico and Africa respectively.

Marigold Wine

According to the seventeenth-century herbalist and physician, Nicholas Culpeper, the flowers of the sunny Marigold made drink that was 'a comforter of the heart and spirits,' so this wine should bring some cheerfulness into the day.

You will need

* 1.7 liters (3 pints) Marigold petals, loosely packed
* 1 lemon
* 2 oranges
* 1 Campden tablet, crushed
* 4.5 liters (1 gallon) water
* 1.2 kg (2½ lb) sugar
* yeast and nutrient
* 225 g (8 oz) sultanas, chopped
* 5 ml (1 teaspoon) grape tannin

Method

1   Thinly pare the lemon and oranges, and put the parings with the Marigold petals into a fermenting bin with the crushed Campden tablet.
2   Bring 3.5 liters (6 pints) of the water to a boil and pour it over the flowers, stir, cover and leave to steep for 24 hours.
3   Heat the remaining 1 liter (2 pints) of water to about 27°C (80°F) and stir it into the sugar in a separate container. Stir to dissolve the sugar, then add the yeast. Leave for 15 minutes.
4   Pour the yeasted sugar syrup into the fermenting bin, stirring well, then stir in the sultanas, the juice of the lemon and oranges, and the tannin.
5   Cover and keep in a warm place for five days, stirring twice daily.
6   Strain into a demijohn, fit the airlock and leave in a warm place to continue fermenting, racking as a sediment forms.
7   When the wine is clear and fermentation has finished, bottle, cork, and label. Store for four months before opening.

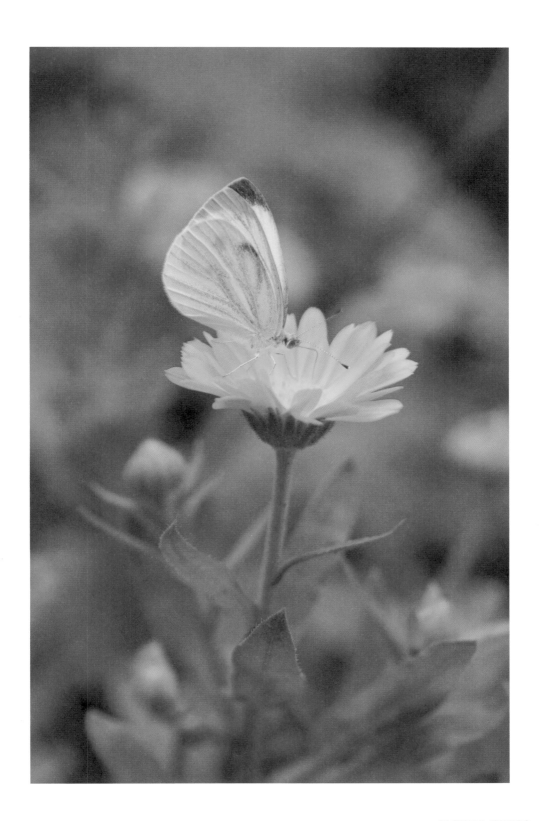

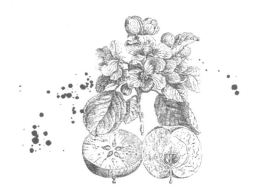

FRUIT WINES

Most fruits – wild or cultivated – make good wine, with their acids (detectable by a sharp taste), sugars, juices, and good flavors and colors. Tannin is usually present to some degree, but different acids dominate in different fruits, and sometimes the acid content needs to be balanced with citric or other acids. With sweet pears and cherries, blueberries and other sweet fruits, the acid content is low and must be boosted. The main difficulty with fruits can be the presence of pectins, which cloud the wine, so for many it is vital to use a pectic enzyme to counter this. Fruits can be used whole, as they are, but windfalls must be cleaned of soil, and other fruits should be quickly washed unless particularly delicate. When paring lemons and oranges for their zest, scrub them first and take care to exclude all the pith, which gives a bitter taste. Always use fruit that is ripe and in good condition, or cut away damaged parts of windfall apples, pears, and other orchard fruit. Frozen, dried or canned fruits can be used as well as fresh. All fruits are normally used uncooked.

Apple
see Crab Apple, page 98

Apricot
Prunus armeniaca

So well known, this summer fruit needs no describing. Apricots originate from China, and are generally orchard or garden fruit, though in very warm places they can escape to be found in the wild. In northern Europe and other cooler climates, you will need the shelter of a sunny wall if you want to grow your own. The plants can be grown as unpruned bushes, reaching about 2.4 m (8 ft) high and spreading to 3.5 m (12 ft), but are often trained into a fan shape. Blossom appears in late winter or early spring and must be protected from frost or the fruit will not set.

You'll find it in southern areas of Europe and other parts of the world with a favorable climate, where you may be able to pick your own Apricots at a fruit farm – but for most people the time to use them will be when there is a glut of imported fruit in shops and markets and large quantities can be bought quite cheaply.

Apricot Wine

Apricots make a medium-sweet white wine. The recipe is adaptable since fresh, dried, or canned fruit can be used and a sweeter version can also be made, which is delicious sipped with dessert. When using fresh Apricots, select ripe fruits that are not too soft.

You will need
* 1.8 kg (4 lb) fresh Apricots or 450 g (1 lb) dried
* 10 ml (2 teaspoons) acid blend
* 10 ml (2 teaspoons) grape tannin
* 4.5 liters (1 gallon) water
* 1.3 kg (3 lb) sugar
* 2.5 ml (½ teaspoon) pectic enzyme powder
* yeast and nutrient
* finings (optional, see Method)
* 1 vitamin C tablet, crushed
* 1 Campden tablet, crushed (for Sweet Wine, see page 80)

Method

1 Remove the stones from the Apricots and crush the fruit in a fermenting bin. Add the acid blend and grape tannin. Keep covered while you bring the water to a boil.

2 Stir in the sugar and pour on the boiling water. Stir to make sure that the sugar is completely dissolved, then cover and leave to cool.

3 When the pulp has cooled to 24°C (75°F), add the pectic enzyme powder and the wine yeast, cover again, and leave to ferment for about six days, stirring twice daily.

4 Strain off the liquid, pressing gently to get all the juice, then transfer it to a demijohn and fit the airlock. Put it in a warm place for fermentation to continue.

5 Rack as the wine clears and sediment forms. Finings may be needed to help this wine to clear (following the instructions on the packet).

6 When the wine is clear and fermentation has stopped, add a crushed vitamin C tablet to prevent discoloration. Bottle, cork, and label. Store for a year before drinking.

Note

* For canned Apricots, use approximately the same weight as fresh, including the syrup from the can.

Sweet Apricot Wine

A sweeter version of this wine can be made by adding sugar syrup to taste at the bottling stage. Use a mix of two parts sugar to one part hot water, dissolve well, and cool before using. Also add a crushed Campden tablet in order to prevent further fermentation.

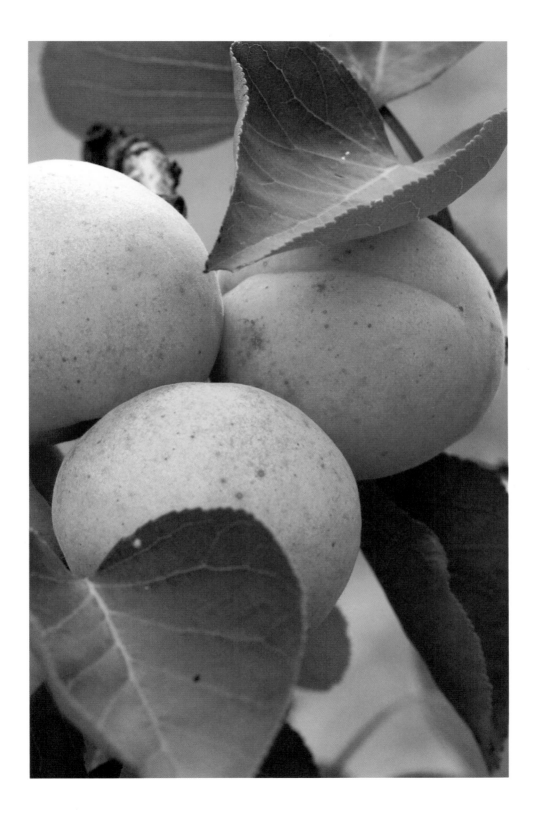

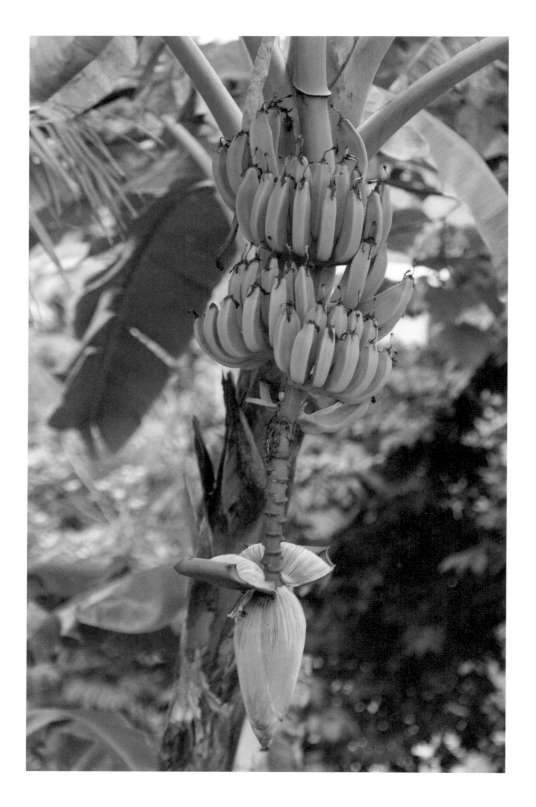

Banana

Musa **species**

Bananas are tropical fruits that come from areas such as Southeast Asia, North Africa, and Central and South America, and are now grown particularly in the West Indies as a crop for the world market, available throughout the year. Large, evergreen herbaceous plants, with extremely big, broad leaves, their fruits are so well known as to need no description here. They come in many sizes, and in purple and red varieties as well as the familiar yellow ones.

This is not a plant you will harvest on your Sunday walk, and in temperate regions you will need a large glasshouse and dedication if you want to grow your own. Nevertheless Bananas are sometimes sold very cheaply at the end of the day in markets and supermarkets, and you may wish to try making a more unusual wine. Over-ripe Bananas from the fruit bowl can also be put to good use this way.

Body building Bananas and Banana skins are rich in minerals and can be used to add body to any wine. While the less ripe fruits are very starchy, which can cause problems, using their skins alone is unproblematic.

Banana Wine

The high levels of starch in Bananas can cause the wine to be cloudy, or make it very slow to clear. For this reason a starch-clearing enzyme is used in the recipe. Since the starch is converted to sugar during the ripening process, over-ripe fruits are best for wine.

You will need
* 1.8 kg (4 lb) ripe Bananas or 225 g (8 oz) dried
* 2.5 ml (½ teaspoon) grape tannin (optional, see Method)
* 450 g (1 lb) raisins, chopped
* 1.3 kg (3 lb) sugar
* 5 ml (1 teaspoon) starch enzyme
* 20 ml (4 teaspoons) acid blend
* 4.5 liters (1 gallon) water
* yeast and nutrient
* 1 vitamin C tablet

Method

1   Slice the Bananas into a fermenting bin with four Banana skins (also sliced) or the grape tannin. Add the chopped raisins and mix in the sugar, starch enzyme and acid blend.

2   Bring the water to a boil, pour it over the fruit, stir well to ensure that the sugar is dissolved, and allow to cool. Add the yeast when the temperature is 21–24° C (70–75°F).

3   Cover and leave to ferment for a week, stirring thoroughly twice daily.

4   Strain into a demijohn and fit the airlock. Leave the jar standing in a warm place to ferment.

5   Rack as required, first after about a month, then every three months until the wine is clear. (This can take up to a year.)

6   When the wine is completely clear and fermentation has stopped, add a crushed vitamin C tablet to prevent the wine from browning. Bottle, cork, and label. Store the wine for ten months.

Notes

*   If you have a few skins from firm Bananas available, use these in preference to black ones in Step 1. Tannin should not be needed if the skins are used.

*   If the wine obstinately fails to clear, finings can be used (following the packet instructions).

Blackberry
Rubus fruticosus
also known as Bramble, Briar

Most of us have enjoyed Blackberry picking at some time in our lives, and this European native is a favorite fruit for gathering on country rambles. The fruits mature in late summer and into the autumn, from white or pinkish flowers on the prickly bushes, which often spread themselves over other shrubs or form dense thickets. Even the leaves, which turn to reddish-purple in the autumn, have tiny prickles of their own, while the almost black fruit has deep-red, staining juices. The plant grows in all the temperate regions but thrives particularly well in the British Isles.

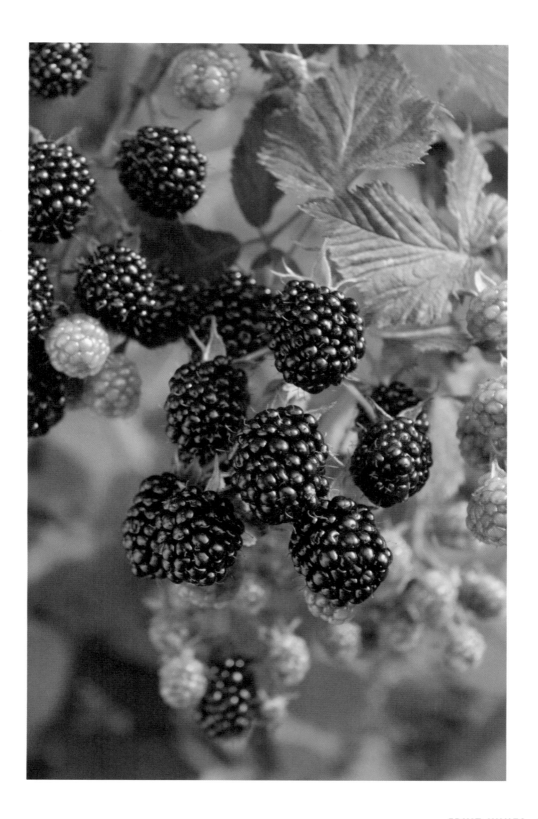

For gathering Blackberries, take a walking stick to pull the branches down, and put the fruit in rigid punnets, bowls, or boxes – not in plastic bags where they will be squashed and bruised. Gather ripe fruits, which are purple and juicy and pull away easily from the stalks, but add a few that are still firm and red for their acidity. Very ripe fruit should be eaten on the spot.

You'll find it growing in hedgerows and beside country roads, on waste ground and neglected sites, by paths and cycle tracks, on commons, and near to railway embankments.

Ancient wisdom The Ancient Greeks used Blackberries as a treatment for gout. Blackberry juice is now known to have an astringent effect and is good for upset stomachs, as well as being a remedy for sore throats and rich in vitamin C.

Blackberry Wine

This makes a beautifully tinted red wine that retains the hedgerow fruit aroma. The color of the wine is fragile, and it needs to be protected from the light. The berries should be used when freshly picked, or frozen at once for later use.

You will need
* 1.8–2.3 kg (4–5 lb) Blackberries
* 1.3 kg (3 lb) sugar
* 4.5 liters (1 gallon) boiling water
* 5 ml (1 teaspoon) acid blend
* 2.5 ml (½ teaspoon) pectic enzyme powder
* yeast and nutrient (see Note, opposite)

Method

1 Crush the fruit in a fermenting bin and add the sugar. Pour on the boiling water and stir well to make sure that the sugar dissolves. Cover and cool to 21–24°C (70–75°F).

2 Add the remaining ingredients, stir, and cover. Leave to ferment for up to a week, stirring daily and pushing down the cap that rises to the surface.

3 Strain, pressing the pulp gently to extract all the juice.

4 Transfer the liquid to a demijohn and fit the airlock. Keep in a warm place while fermentation continues, racking as needed (roughly once after three weeks and again after three months).

5 When fermentation has stopped and the wine is clear, bottle, cork, and label. Store for a year before drinking.

Notes

* Use berries gathered on a dry day. Spreading them out on a plate should encourage any insects to make their exit, as washing them will waste some of their precious juices.

* Burgundy yeast can be used, if available.

* To preserve the color, ferment the wine in a dark glass demijohn, or tape brown parcel paper around the jar to keep the light away. Store the finished wine in dark bottles.

Blackcurrant
Ribes nigrum
also known as Currants, Quinsy Berries

This blue-black summer fruit is seldom found in the wild, though the plants are native to much of Europe as well as northern and central Asia. With their fairly short season and brief 'shelf life,' Blackcurrants are also no longer widely available to buy. Yet Currant bushes can be grown quite easily in ordinary garden soil, sheltered from the wind, and well fed with manure or garden compost. There are also pick-your-own farms where this crop can be found.

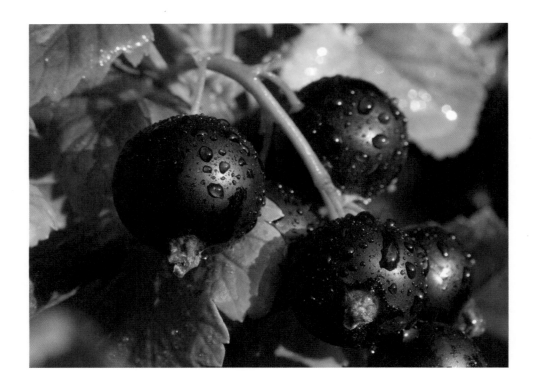

Hardy and clump-forming, the bushes are 1–1.5 m (3½–5 ft) high. Fairly insignificant spring flowers develop into small round fruits that hang in bunches from among the large three- to five-lobed leaves. The leaves are matt-green and when crushed give off the same strong scent as the berries. The fruits are borne on stems put up the previous year, and cutting out the old stems in winter encourages the plant to keep producing new ones.

Blackcurrants are a wonderful source of vitamin C and excellent for jam and jelly making, but also make a very good country wine. Frozen Blackcurrants can be used for this, and are available all year.

You'll find it occasionally growing wild in banks and woodland edges, where the soil is moist. It is best to pick your own at fruit farms or grow a bush yourself. Pick the whole sprigs, preferably by cutting them off with scissors

Blackcurrant Wine

This recipe makes a lovely sweet wine that keeps the taste and bouquet of the fruit. Freezing the fruit first helps to break down the pectin in the Currants, but fresh fruit can be used. Strip the fruits from their stems using a fork before freezing or using fresh.

You will need

* 1.3 kg (3 lb) Blackcurrants, fresh or frozen
* 4.5 liters (1 gallon) water
* 1 Campden tablet, crushed
* 5 ml (1 teaspoon) pectic enzyme powder
* yeast and nutrient
* 1.3 kg (3 lb) sugar

Method

1 Put the prepared Currants in a fermenting bin and crush them with a wooden spoon or rolling pin. Bring the water to a boil and pour it over the fruits.
2 Cover and leave to cool, then stir in the crushed Campden tablet and the pectic enzyme powder. Cover again and leave to steep for 24 hours, stirring once or twice.
3 Activate the yeast (see page 35). Stir the sugar into the bin, stirring until the sugar is dissolved, then add the activated yeast.
4 Cover and leave to ferment for about five days, stirring well and pushing down the cap once or twice a day.
5 Strain off the liquid, making sure you extract as much as possible, and transfer it to a demijohn. Fit the airlock and ferment in a warm place, racking as required.
6 When fermentation has ceased, siphon the wine into dark bottles, cork, and label. Store for a minimum of six months.

Notes

* Blackcurrants are high in pectin, so the pectic enzyme is essential, especially when fresh Currants are used. The amount used can be reduced for frozen fruit.
* The finished wine should be a little like Port and can be served in the same way.

Blueberry
Vaccinium corymbosum
also known as Heathland Berry, Highbush Blueberry
Akin to the native American wild Blueberry, these tasty fruits are now increasingly available in Europe. Still rather expensive to buy, they are not too difficult to grow – provided you can meet their requirement for an acid, well-drained soil (this is essential). They also need a fairly cool, moist climate and some sun (though they tolerate partial shade). Reaching a height of about 1.5 m (5 ft), they can be grown in tubs to give them the soil and situation that they need.

Blueberries are a little slow to get going, but a two- to three-year-old bush will begin to reward your patience with a summer crop of the now familiar blue berries with their blue-grey bloom and delicious sweet flavor, ripening before the leaves turn red.

The fruits store well, and are good to eat raw, but even so it is worth putting some aside for Blueberry Wine.

Blueberry Wine
Blueberries have a good deal of natural sweetness, so less sugar is needed in this wine. Raisins give roundness to the flavor and lemon juice supplies the acid. Huckleberries, where they are available, can replace the Blueberries.

You will need
* 1 kg (2 lb) Blueberries
* 450 g (1 lb) raisins, chopped
* 1 or 2 Campden tablets, crushed (see Note on page 92)
* 4.5 liters (1 gallon) water
* 1 lemon, squeezed
* 2.5 ml (½ teaspoon) pectic enzyme powder
* 1 kg (2 lb) sugar
* yeast and nutrient
* sugar syrup (optional, see Method)

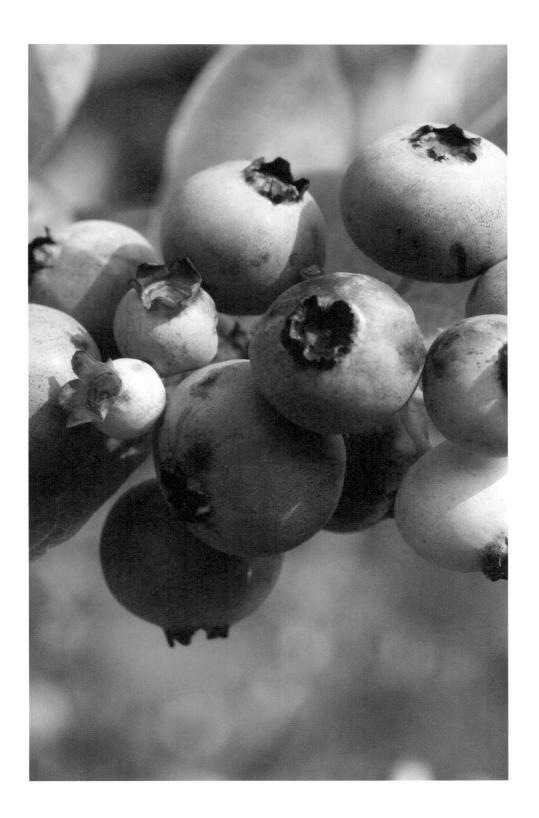

Method

1 Crush the fruit in a fermenting bin and stir in the chopped raisins and a crushed Campden tablet. Boil 3.5 liters (6 pints) of the water, pour it over the fruit and stir well.

2 Allow to cool, then add the lemon juice and pectic enzyme powder. Cover and leave to steep for 24 hours, stirring once or twice.

3 Put the sugar into a large container. Boil the remaining 1 liter (2 pints) of water, pour it onto the sugar and stir well. When the sugar is dissolved pour the syrup into the bin and add the yeast. Cover and leave to ferment for five or six days, stirring twice daily.

4 Strain off the liquid, pressing to extract all the juice, transfer it to a demijohn, and fit the airlock. Put in a warm place to ferment.

5 Rack as required as the fermentation proceeds (about once after three weeks and once again after three months).

6 When fermentation has ceased and the wine has completely cleared, bottle it, cork, and label. Store the wine for one year.

Note

* If you prefer a sweeter wine, add a little sugar syrup to taste (two parts sugar to one part warm water, well dissolved and allowed to cool) before bottling. Stir in a crushed Campden tablet to prevent more fermentation.

Bullace

Prunus domestica subsp. *insititia*

also known as Bullace Plum, Bullums, Damson Plum, Wild Damson

Smaller than Damsons and larger than Sloes, but similar to both, Bullaces were once widely grown in orchards throughout both Europe and North America, as well as in southwest Asia, before larger, sweeter fruit usurped them. The fruits are rounded, bluish-black in color, and have a white or purple bloom. They grow from thorny branches, and the plant itself makes a tall shrub or small tree 1.8–4.5 m (6–15 ft) high. The pure white blossom was known to country people as Bully-blooms and appears in mid-spring, just as the leaves are breaking. The leaves are long and tooth-edged, and take on a leathery thickness as they age.

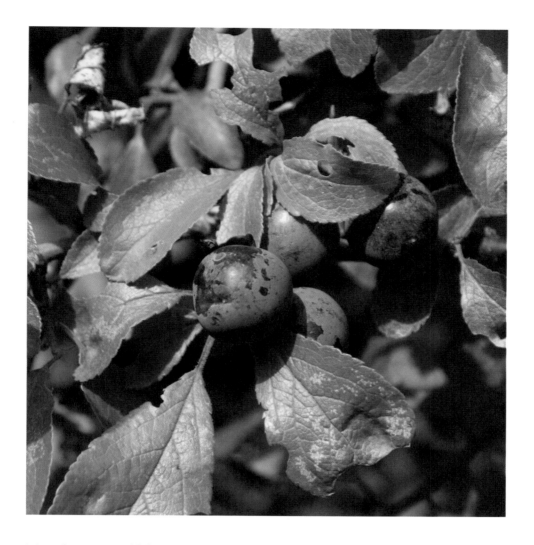

The plants are self-fertile and crop heavily in a good year, so there is plentiful harvest from one bush or tree. The fruit ripens in early autumn. It is firm to the touch and very sharp in flavor, though less so after the autumn frosts, but makes an excellent wine.

You'll find it infrequently, growing alone in hedges and among the shrubs on pastureland and sometimes in old gardens. It is still possible to buy a Bullace plant to grow in the garden, but most people prefer to cultivate a sweeter, juicier type of plum when space is limited.

Bullace Wine

If you can get hold of Bullaces at all, you can get them in plenty. Keep some aside for making this fruity wine, which will glint nicely in the glass. The fruit has a lot of natural acidity and is best not picked until the first frosts have softened it.

You will need

* 1.8 kg (4 lb) Bullaces
* 225 g (8 oz) raisins, chopped
* 4.5 liters (1 gallon) water
* 5 ml (1 teaspoon) pectic enzyme powder
* 1 Campden tablet, crushed
* yeast and nutrient
* 1.3 kg (3 lb) sugar

Method

1 Put the Bullaces in a large container or fermenting bin and crush them against the sides with a wooden spoon or rolling pin. Add the raisins, boil the water, and pour it over the fruit.
2 Allow to cool, then stir in the pectic enzyme powder and crushed Campden tablet. Cover, and steep for four days, stirring thoroughly twice daily. Activate the yeast at the end of this period (see page 35).
3 Strain the Bullace liquid onto the sugar in a fermenting bin, stir well, and when the sugar is fully dissolved add the yeast. Cover again and allow to ferment in a warm place for about a week, continuing to stir as before.
4 Siphon into a demijohn, fit the airlock, and continue with the fermentation in a warm place, racking once or twice as required.
5 If possible, transfer the cleared wine into a second demijohn when fermentation has stopped and bung it up completely. Store in a cool, dark environment to mature for a year, then bottle, cork, and label. Store for a further year or two to enjoy the wine at its best. (Alternatively, bottle, cork, and label the wine and store it for a minimum of two years.)

Plums (*Prunus domestica* varieties)

Plums are broadly similar to Bullaces, and have gradually taken over from them as orchard and garden fruit. Purple-, orange-, and yellow-hued Plums have been developed and some escape from gardens into the countryside and form hybrids.

All sorts of Plums, whether homegrown, store-bought, or found growing in the wild, can be used to make fruit wine following the Bullace recipe. Different Plums will produce wines of different qualities and color. The well-known 'Victoria' Plum produces a rosé wine, while the sharper-tasting purple cooking Plums produce a golden yellow one, and the amber yellow 'Golden Drop' will produce a paler yellow wine. You may enjoy experimenting with different varieties and different ratios of fruit to sugar, adding lemon juice or acid blend for sweet dessert Plums.

Cherry

Prunus avium (European); *Prunus serotina* (North American)
also known as Gean, Mazzard, Wild Cherry (European); Black Cherry, Mountain Black Cherry, Rum Cherry, Wild Black Cherry (North American)
Wild Cherry trees are native to Britain, most of Europe and western Asia. A similar tree grows extensively in North America from southern Quebec and Ontario to Texas and central Florida, with populations in Arizona and New Mexico.

The trees tend to produce acid, sharp-tasting fruit, and grow to a height of 12 m (40 ft) or more, with spread to match. Until not so many decades ago, the only Cherry trees for gardens were likewise inconveniently tall, except for a few that also bore sharp-tasting fruit. New rootstocks now enable much smaller trees to be grown, and self-fertile, sweet varieties are available as compact trees for the average garden.

Shiny red or blackish-red Cherries bunched on their woody stems are well known. The trees themselves have stout branches and glossy reddish-brown bark banded with peeling strips and areas of pale brown breathing pores. The new spring leaves are a delightful bronze and begin to open just after the ephemeral clouds of delicate white blossom. The Wild Cherry is quite a common tree, but the rapid fading of its blossom perhaps makes it less noticeable than it deserves to be.

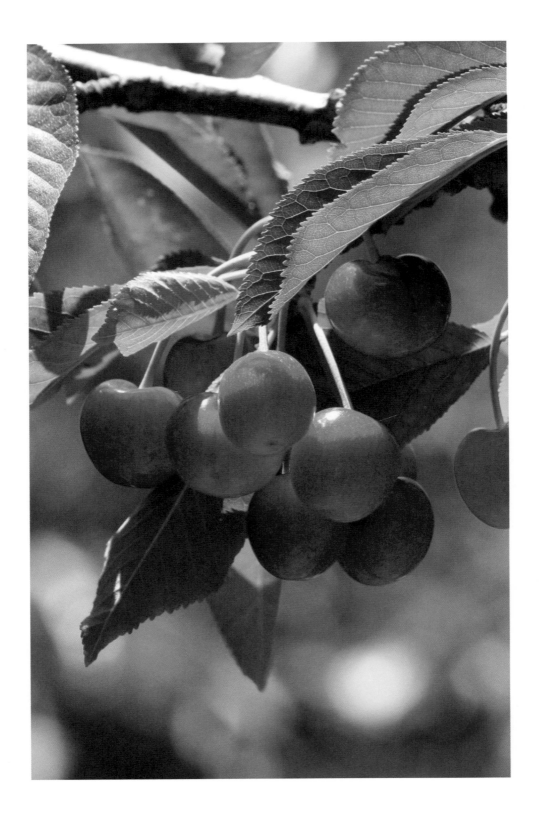

You'll find it in woodland and hedgerows, particularly where the soil is limey or chalky. The Cherries are quickly taken by the birds, and it is more likely that you will be using garden or commercially grown Cherries for your wine.

Cherry Wine

A good Cherry Wine is smooth and medium-sweet, light but with full Cherry flavors. The color depends on the type of Cherries used. A blend of fruits can be used, or just one type, and you will need to use more Cherries if all are sweet.

You will need
* 1.8 kg (4 lb) sour Cherries or 2.7 kg (6 lb) sweet Cherries
* 15 ml (3 teaspoons) acid blend
* 2 Campden tablets, crushed (see Note, page 98)
* 2.5 ml (½ teaspoon) grape tannin
* 1.2 kg (2½ lb) sugar
* 4.5 liters (1 gallon) hot water
* yeast and nutrient
* 2.5 ml (½ teaspoon) pectic enzyme powder (5 ml/1 teaspoon for sour Cherries)
* sugar syrup (optional, see Method)
* 1 vitamin C tablet, crushed

Method
1   Wash the fruit and reject any Cherries that are unsound, or over- or under-ripe. Remove the stems and any leaves. Lightly crush the Cherries in a fermenting bin and add the acid blend, a crushed Campden tablet, and the grape tannin.
2   Stir in the sugar, pour on the hot water, and stir well to dissolve the sugar.
3   Cover and leave to steep for 24 hours. Activate the yeast at the end of this period (see page 35).
4   Add the pectic enzyme powder and yeast, cover, and leave to ferment for about five days, stirring daily and pushing down the Cherries as they rise.
5   Strain off the liquid, pressing the pulp to extract all the juices. Transfer to a demijohn and fit the airlock. Leave in a warm place to ferment for about four months, racking once or twice as the liquid clears.
6   When fermentation has ceased and the wine is clear, add the crushed vitamin C tablet to prevent oxidation and bottle the wine in dark bottles. Cork and label. Store for a year before drinking.

Notes

* It would be impractical to remove the Cherry stones, but take care not to break them when you crush the fruit.
* Some winemakers add a crushed Campden tablet before bottling, as a precaution against the wine fermenting in the bottles.

Sweet Wine For a sweeter wine, add sugar syrup to taste before bottling (two parts sugar, one part hot water, well dissolved and allowed to cool). Add a crushed Campden tablet to prevent further fermentation.

Crab Apple

Malus sylvestris

also known as Crabs, European Apple, Sour Grabs

Crab Apple trees are native to most of Europe and southwest Asia, and are now found growing wild in many parts of North America. The trees grow to a height of 7.5 m (25 ft) and bear pink-flushed, lightly scented apple blossom in spring, followed by late summer fruit. This can be produced in profusion in a good year, and the small Apples are greenish-yellow in color with a very sharp taste, often ripening to a redder shade. The leaves are simple and roundish, with bluntly toothed edges, mid- to dark green, and usually downy.

Many wild Apple trees are garden escapes, with larger, sweeter fruit, and true Crab Apples can be distinguished by the sourness of the fruit and by their shape – with a depression at both ends of the fruit. Fallen Crab Apples and any other Apples, wild or from the garden, can be used for wine.

You'll find it growing in light woodland, hedgerows, and open ground, usually in isolation. Spot your tree and go back after a windy day in late summer or early autumn to pick up the harvest.

Old ancestor The Crab Apple is the ancestor of all our dessert Apples, of which there are now thousands of different varieties. Archaeological evidence shows that the fruits were used for cooking in prehistoric times.

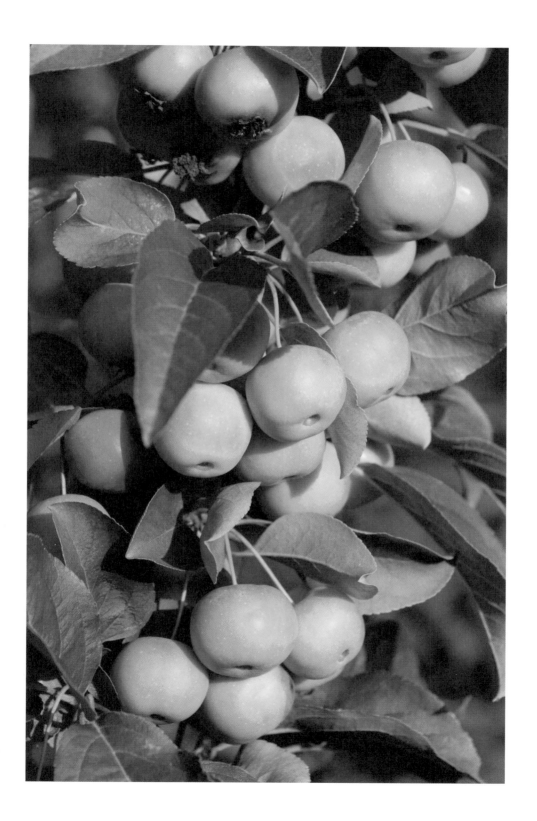

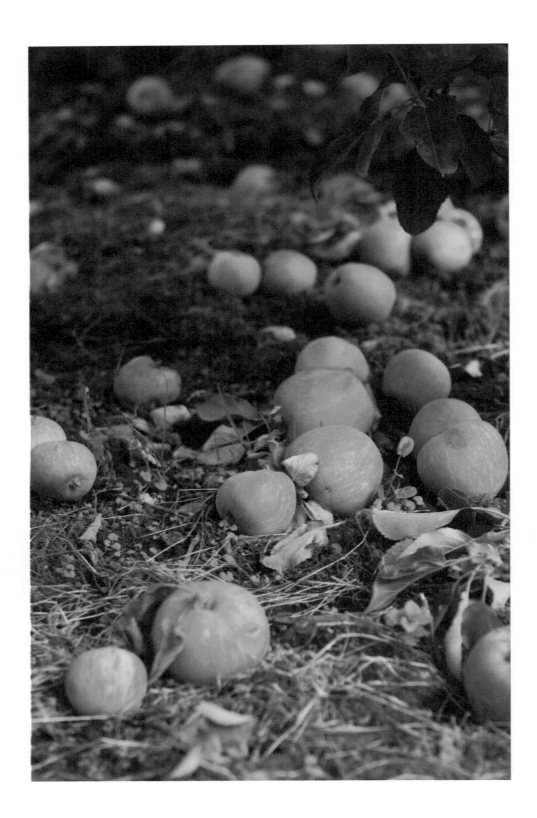

Apple Wine

This traditional country wine is a wonderful way of putting windfall or surplus Apples to good use, and a mixture of varieties can be used. The Crab Apple variation appears on page 102. Both make a pleasantly light white wine.

You will need

* 4.5–5.5 kg (10–12 lb) Apples
* 1 Campden tablet, crushed
* 2.5 ml (½ teaspoon) pectic enzyme powder
* 4.5 liters (1 gallon) water
* yeast and nutrient
* 1.2 kg (2½) lb sugar
* 1 vitamin C tablet, crushed

Method

1 Rinse the Apples and inspect them for damage, cutting off any bruised or damaged parts but otherwise leaving them whole.

2 Chop the Apples roughly into small pieces and put them into a fermenting bin with the crushed Campden tablet. Crushing the fruit will help to extract maximum juices and flavor. Add the pectic enzyme powder.

3 Pour the water over the Apples. Cover and steep for 24 hours, stirring well once or twice.

4 Activate the yeast at the end of this time (see page 35).

5 Add the sugar to the bin and stir well to dissolve it, then add the yeast. Cover again, and leave in a warm place to ferment for about five more days, stirring firmly once or twice daily.

6 Strain off into a demijohn, extracting as much liquid as possible. Fit the airlock, move to a warm place, and carry on fermenting, racking as necessary. This may take from one to three months.

7 When the wine is clear and fermentation has ceased, add a vitamin C tablet to prevent discoloration, then siphon off into bottles. Cork, label, and store for at least six months, but preferably a year.

Note

* If your Apples are all very sweet, add the juice of two lemons with the yeast to give acidity.

Crab Apple Wine

You will need
* 2.7 kg (6 lb) Crab Apples
* 450 g (1 lb) raisins
* 1.2 kg (2½ lb) sugar
* 1 Campden tablet, crushed
* 4.5 liters (1 gallon) water
* yeast and nutrient
* 2.5 ml (½ teaspoon) pectic enzyme powder
* 1 vitamin C tablet, crushed
* finings (optional, see Note below)

Method
1 Cut up or crush the Crab Apples, chop the raisins, and put them both into a fermenting bin together with the sugar and the crushed Campden tablet. Stir well together.
2 Heat the water, and pour it over the blended ingredients. Stir again to dissolve the sugar.
3 When the contents of the bin have cooled to 21°C (70°F), add the yeast and the pectic enzyme powder, cover, and leave to ferment for five to six days, stirring daily.
4 Strain off the liquid, gently pressing the solids to extract it all, and transfer to a demijohn. Fit the airlock and leave in a warm place to ferment. Rack the wine once or twice as it clears.
5 When the wine has cleared and fermentation has stopped, add a vitamin C tablet to prevent discoloration, then siphon off into bottles, cork well, and label. Store for a year before drinking.

Note
* This wine may need to be cleared with finings, following the instructions on the packet.

Damson

Prunus damascena

Native to the Middle East, Damsons were reputedly brought into northern Europe by returning crusaders. Another theory states that they were introduced to England much earlier by the Romans. Certainly there is archaeological evidence that the Romans knew and used the fruit. The Damson was introduced to the American colonies by early English settlers.

Once much cultivated for use in cooking and for making jams or jelly, Damsons are now just as likely to be found growing wild, forming bushes up to 3.5 m (12 ft) high or small trees up to a height of 7.5 m (25 ft) that are covered with airy white blossom in early spring – somewhat later than the Blackthorn (Sloes) and Plums. The late summer fruits are a deep dark purple, often with a blue bloom. Similar in shape to Bullaces, but a little larger, softer, and slightly sweeter (though still tart), they are perfect for making country wine.

You'll find them growing wild in woods or thickets and hedges, especially near the site of an old orchard. Damsons crop abundantly, ripening in late summer or early autumn, and should be picked on the point of ripeness. The easiest way to gather them is to scoop them up from the ground as soon as they begin to fall.

Growing Damsons Damsons prefer heavy, loamy, well-drained soil, but will grow even in cold and windswept gardens. Hardier than plums, and flowering later, they are less vulnerable to frost and tolerate both exposed and fairly shady conditions that would be less than ideal for plums, putting up with higher rainfall and less sun. They can even be grown as windbreaks, should you need one.

Self-fertile Damsons for the garden
* early spring – 'Merryweather'
* mid-spring – 'Bradley's King'
* mid- to late spring – 'Prune' (aka 'Shropshire')

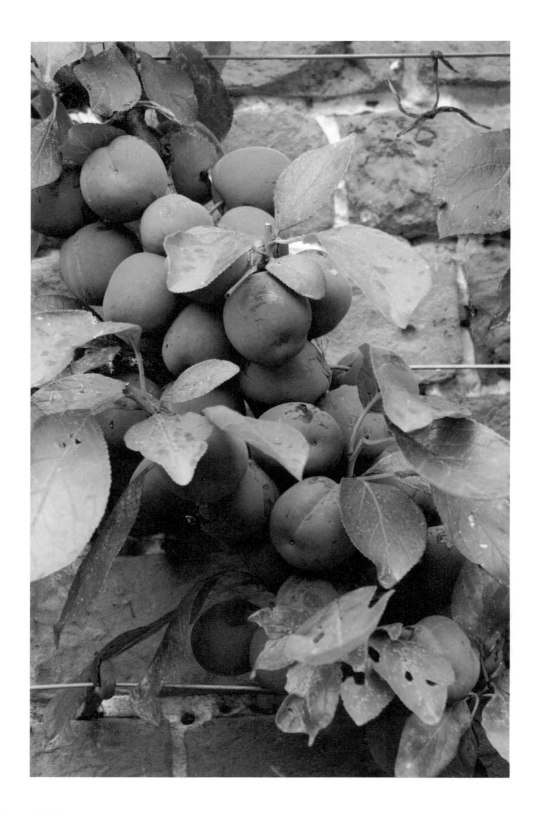

Antique purple Damsons have been appreciated and cultivated since antiquity. They are thought to have been grown originally in the area around Damascus, in modern-day Syria, reputedly the oldest city in the world. In ancient times, they were used to make a purple dye as well as forming part of the diet.

Damson Wine

This wine has the true country flavor of wild wine. The longer you can wait before drinking it, the better it will be. Damson Wine has a deep purple-red color and is on the dry side, with a fruity richness.

You will need

* 1.3 kg (3 lb) ripe Damsons
* 4.5 liters (1 gallon) water
* 1.3 kg (3 lb) sugar
* 10 ml (2 teaspoons) pectic enzyme powder
* 1 Campden tablet, crushed
* yeast and nutrient

Method

1   Using a very large saucepan or a preserving pan, bring the Damsons to the boil in the water, skimming off the stones as they rise to the surface. Simmer gently until the fruits are tender but still whole.
2   Strain off the liquid into a fermenting bin, retaining the fruits in the strainer (they can be used for jam or other recipes).
3   Pour the sugar into the bin and stir well to make sure the sugar is all dissolved. Cover and allow to cool, then add the pectic enzyme powder and crushed Campden tablet.
4   Cover, and keep in a warm place for 24 hours, then add the yeast and allow to ferment for three days, stirring daily.
5   Transfer to a demijohn, fit the airlock, and put the jar in a warm place for fermentation to continue, racking as the wine clears.
6   When fermentation has stopped and the wine is clear, bottle it in dark bottles, cork, and label. Store for at least a year before drinking.

Notes

* Generally very acid, the fruits need no supplementary acid in the recipe but they are rich in pectin and the pectic enzyme is imperative.
* Damson Wine takes time to mature and benefits from being kept in a cool place in a demijohn, well bunged, for a year before you bottle it. The wine will mellow slowly, and rewards patience.

Elderberry
Sambucus nigra

The Elder plant has been described in the Flower Recipes section, as its flowers can be used for fragrant summery wines (see page 66), but the autumn fruits must not be overlooked. With their medicinal properties, as well as the advantage of being so readily available, the berries of the Elder have always been highly valued by country people.

Purple-black when ripe, hanging in round bunches on reddish stems, Elderberries are produced in abundance at the end of summer and in early autumn. The juicy fruits look superficially like small blackcurrants and are so plentiful that they cause the branches to bend under their weight. Birds find them very attractive and often whole bunches will be picked dry – but there will always be some left on the plants for us. The purple-red juices with their strong, fruity scent make one of the best wild wines.

You'll find it in hedgerows, by ponds and streams, in woods and fields. Choose plants growing in the sun and cut off the bunches that look really ripe, or pinch them off with your fingers. The largest berries will, of course, yield most juice.

The habits of rabbits Rabbits often have their warrens in among Elder bushes. The Elders thrive because for some reason the rabbits do not eat them, and the rabbits survive because the Elder roots are not big enough to obstruct the rabbits' burrowing and the shrubs provide plenty of cover.

Cash crop Elder was once grown commercially for making wine, and the juices of the fruits were also added to grape wines to give them color.

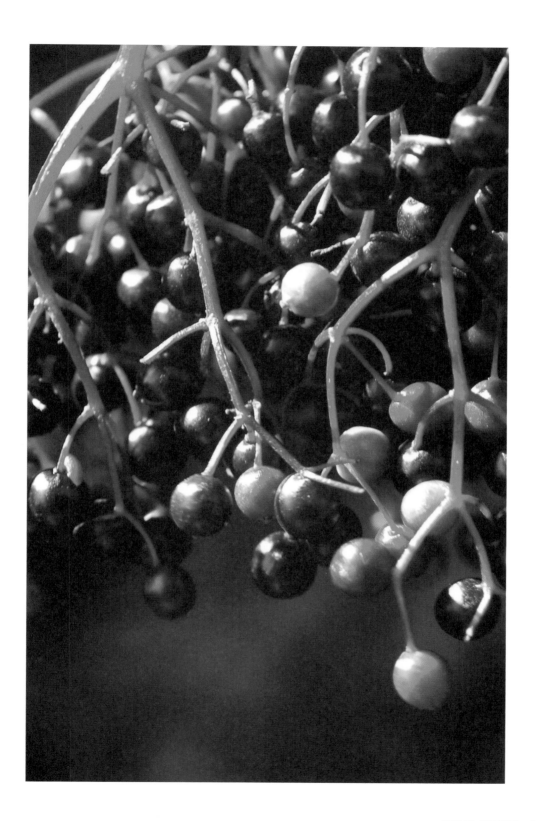

Elderberry Wine

Elderberry Wine is a real old country favorite. Deep dark red and semi-sweet, it makes a warming winter drink the year after bottling, and matures with storing. Perfect for sipping by the fire, it can also be drunk hot to cure a feverish cold.

You will need

* 1.6 kg (3½ lb) Elderberries
* 450 g (1 lb) mixed raisins and sultanas, chopped
* 4.5 liters (1 gallon) boiling water
* 1 lemon, squeezed
* yeast and nutrient
* 1.3 kg (3 lb) sugar

Method

1   Strip the Elderberries from their stems, using a fork, and mash them in a fermenting bin with the chopped dried fruit. Pour the boiling water over the fruits and allow to cool.

2   When the mixture is at blood heat, add the juice of the lemon and the yeast, cover, and stand in a warm place to ferment for about a week, stirring once or twice daily and pushing down the cap that rises to the surface.

3   Strain off the solids and add the sugar to the liquid, stirring to make sure it is completely dissolved, then transfer the liquid to a demijohn. Fit the airlock and leave the wine to continue fermenting in a warm place. Rack as the sediment forms.

4   When fermentation has ceased, transfer the wine to another demijohn and fit a bung. Leave it to mature in a cool place for six months, then bottle, cork, and label. Store for a further six months. Alternatively, bottle the wine at once, and store for a year.

Notes

* In this method, the yeast begins to feed on the sweet vine fruit and the sugar is added at a later stage.
* This recipe can be made with 225 g (8 oz) of dried Elderberries. The fresh fruit can also be used frozen.
* This wine will probably need to be racked at least three times, and may continue fermenting for several months.

Gooseberry

Ribes uva-crispa

also known as English Gooseberry, European Gooseberry, Feaberry, Goosegog

Gooseberries are native to a large area of Europe, from the south to Scandinavia, and also in north Africa. They grow wild in parts of North America as well, where they have escaped from gardens. Normally they are not found in large numbers, except in rare locations.

The veined fruits are round or oval, and usually covered in hairs. Green with a yellow or sometimes reddish-brown tinge, they hang among the leaves in small clusters, ripening in early to mid-summer. The deciduous bushes are spiny and branching, and grow to a height of about 1 m (3½ ft). The small leaves are matt green, with three or five lobes, and the fruits develop from small greenish-colored flowers that appear in spring and early summer.

Despite being indigenous, Gooseberries are mainly cultivated in gardens and fruit farms. They are often in short supply in the shops these days, but there are still farms in the countryside where you can pick your own fruit, and one Gooseberry bush in the garden will fruit abundantly in a good year. Many varieties are available for garden cultivation, from sharp-tasting, firm, thick-skinned culinary fruits (for cooking) to the larger, sweet-tasting, thinner-skinned dessert (sweet) kinds. Most are easy to grow and not fussy as to soil, though all benefit from care and attention.

You'll find it occasionally, growing in relatively damp and shady places, by streams and waterways. More often, garden Gooseberry bushes get sown by the birds, and can be found near hedges and in light woodland close to gardens.

Gooseberry Wine

The main recipe on page 111 makes a dry, crisp white wine. Dessert Gooseberries can be used to make a sweeter wine with a stronger Gooseberry flavor, and the recipe can also be adapted to produce a Champagne-type sparkling wine, good for celebrations (for these variations, see page 112).

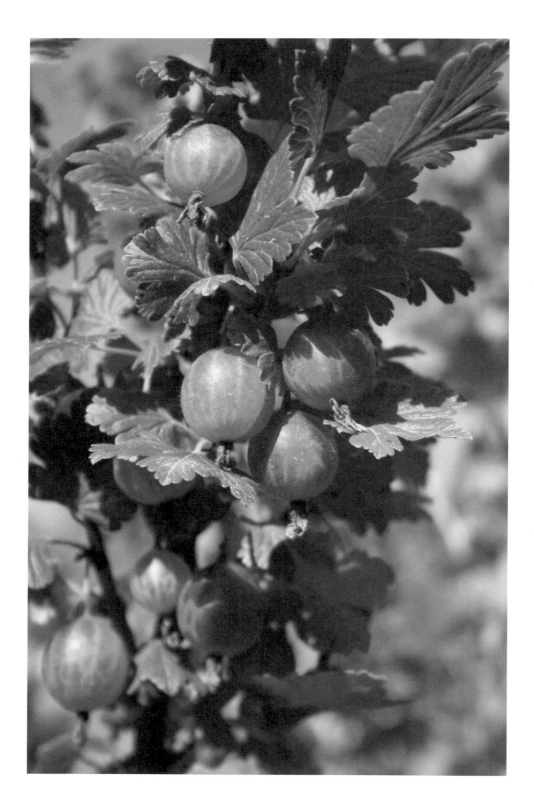

You will need

* 1.8 kg (4 lb) cooking Gooseberries
* 2 Campden tablets, crushed (see Method)
* 4.5 liters (1 gallon) water
* 5 ml (1 teaspoon) acid blend
* 2.5 ml (½ teaspoon) grape tannin
* 2.5 ml (½ teaspoon) pectic enzyme powder
* 1.2 kg (2½ lb) sugar
* yeast and nutrient
* sugar syrup (optional, see Method)

Method

1   Rinse the Gooseberries in a colander (no need to top and tail). Put them into a fermenting bin, crushing them against the sides to get the juices running.
2   Stir in a crushed Campden tablet, bring 3.5 liters (6 pints) of water to a boil and pour it over the Gooseberries. Stir well, cover, and allow to cool.
3   When cool, add the acid blend, grape tannin, and pectic enzyme powder. Cover and leave to steep for 24 hours, stirring once or twice. At the end of this time, stir in the sugar, stirring well to make sure it is fully dissolved.
4   Boil the remaining 1 liter (2 pints) of water and pour into the bin. Add the yeast, cover, and leave to ferment for four days, stirring twice daily and pressing down the cap that comes up to the surface.
5   Strain off the liquid, pressing gently to extract all the juice, transfer to a demijohn and fit the airlock. Ferment in a warm place, racking once or twice as required.
6   When fermentation has stopped and the wine has completely cleared, transfer it to a storage jar, add one crushed Campden tablet and insert the bung firmly.
7   Store the wine in a cool, dark place for six months, checking it from time to time, and racking if a sediment forms.
8   At the end of this time, bottle, cork, and label the wine. Store for another six months before drinking.

Sweet Gooseberry Wine

If you prefer a sweeter wine, use 1.3 kg (3 lb) sugar in the main recipe, and before bottling add a little sugar syrup (two parts sugar to one part hot water, well dissolved and allowed to cool) to taste. Also mix in a crushed Campden tablet to prevent fermentation in the bottles.

Dessert Gooseberry Wine

To make a sweeter, more Gooseberry-flavored wine, follow the main recipe but use 1.8 kg (4 lb) ripe red dessert Gooseberries and 1.3 kg (3 lb) sugar.

Gooseberry 'Champagne'

The Gooseberries with richest flavor are the yellow kind, and wine from them is like Champagne. To make a sparkling wine, proceed to the end of Step 5, then bottle the wine in strong, Champagne-type bottles and add a small teaspoon of sugar to each bottle. Use purpose-made plastic stoppers and wire them firmly in place. Store the bottles upright in a cool, dark place for six months to a year, checking occasionally that the stoppers are holding firm. Don't worry about the slight sediment that forms at the base of the bottles.

Grapefruit
Citrus × paradisi
also known as Pomelo

For a citrus fruit recipe with Grapefruit, see pages 130–131

Greengage
Prunus domestica **subsp.** *italica*
also known as Gage, Reine Claude

These sweet, green, or greenish-yellow plums were introduced to Britain from France by an English lord, Sir William Gage, a quarter of a century ago. Greengages had been developed in Moissac, southern France, from wild plums themselves originating from Asia Minor. The original Greengages are still found, and many newer Gages are available too. All do best in warmer climates and are ideal for training against a sunny wall.

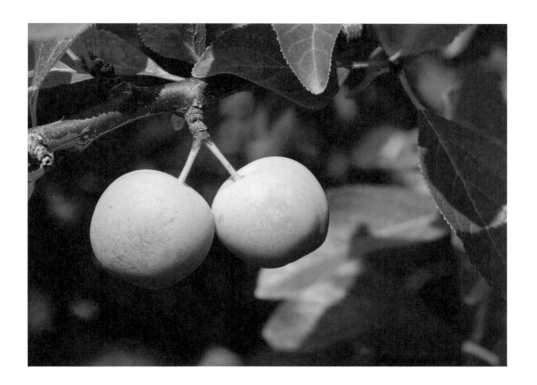

The white blossom in spring develops into fruits that are round and walnut-sized, with a light blue bloom on the thin skins, and clear, almost transparent flesh. The fruit ripens in late summer and plants are available as small bushes or orchard trees ranging from 2.4 to 4.3 m (8–14 ft) in height. Quick growers, they need little pruning unless they are to be wall-grown. Many are self-fertile, so only one is needed. If you grow your own, it may produce a heavy crop in favorable circumstances. The fruits don't keep well, so making wine is a perfect way to use a surplus.

You'll find them in gardens, and occasionally at pick-your-own orchards or for sale as garden produce outside country houses. Gages are available in the shops in late summer, but usually expensive.

Cold comfort Gages are not at home in less than balmy places. More demanding than plums, they need more warmth and shelter. Though they fruit in later summer, most flower early and are vulnerable to cold weather, so the trees will not produce well in places prone to spring frosts. Try growing them only if you have a sunny, sheltered garden.

Presidential plums   Greengages were introduced to North America in the eighteenth century and soon became popular. They were grown in their Virginian plantations by two United States Presidents: George Washington, a keen gardener and plantsman, and Thomas Jefferson. They were also widely grown in the American colonies in the eighteenth and early nineteenth centuries.

Greengage Wine

Greengages make a pleasant light white wine. As with all plums and stone fruit, the stones contain pectin and should not be crushed during the preparation process. The citrus fruits in this recipe add the necessary acidity.

You will need
* 1.8 kg (4 lb) Greengages
* 2 lemons
* 4.5 liters (1 gallon) water
* 1 Campden tablet, crushed
* 1.3 kg (3 lb) sugar
* 1 orange, squeezed
* yeast and nutrient

Method
1   Halve the Greengages into a fermenting bin, catching all the juices. Pare the lemons and add the pared zest to the bin. Bring the water to a boil and pour it over the fruits. Stir and press to extract the juices.
2   Add the crushed Campden tablet, cover, and leave to infuse for two days, stirring once or twice a day.
3   Stir in the sugar, stirring well until it is dissolved. Add the squeezed orange juice and the yeast, cover, and leave to ferment in a warm place for three days, stirring twice daily and pushing down the cap that rises to the surface.
4   Strain off the liquid and transfer it to a demijohn. Fit the airlock and continue fermenting in a warm place, racking as the sediment forms.
5   When the wine is clear and no longer fermenting, bottle, cork, and label. Store for at least six months.

Haw (Hawthorn Fruit)

Crataegus monogyna

also known as Cuckoo's Beads, Pixie Pears

Hawthorns and where to find them growing have been described in the Flower section (see page 72). The fruits or Haws start to develop soon after the blossoms disappear, gradually turning from green to a warm red. When ready to pick, Haws are plump and dark red and look like clusters of tiny apples (to which they are related). Inside, the fruits are mealy, with cream-colored flesh. Each has a single stone (which is what *monogyna* means), and the taste is bitter and astringent – not a fruit for eating raw. These miniature apples are much enjoyed by birds, which also find nesting places in the dense branches. Thanks to them, self-seeded plants soon spread on scrubland, providing shelter for sheep and other animals. Pick whole clusters of the fruits from hedgerows and trees where they are plentiful, and always leave plenty for the local wildlife.

Growing a Hawthorn bush in your garden will attract pollinating insects to the blossoms and birds to the fruits, as well as providing you with your own harvest. To keep it as a bush, trim it regularly, wearing gloves for protection.

Good old ways Hawthorn is a tough and long-lived shrub, and many of the hedges still remaining were planted in the eighteenth century. Though machine-clipped Hawthorn makes a sturdy hedge for farmland, it will not produce flowers and fruit. In contrast, the old practice of hedge laying (whereby the branches are bent down and woven across each other horizontally) encourages blossom, making hedgerows that are rich in Haws that attract and feed birds, woodmice, and other small wild creatures.

Hawthorn Wine

This being a traditional country wine, there are many ways of making it, and the amount of Haws used can be varied. The recipe here should make a fairly dry but fruity white wine. A sparkling version can be made following the method for Gooseberry (see page 111).

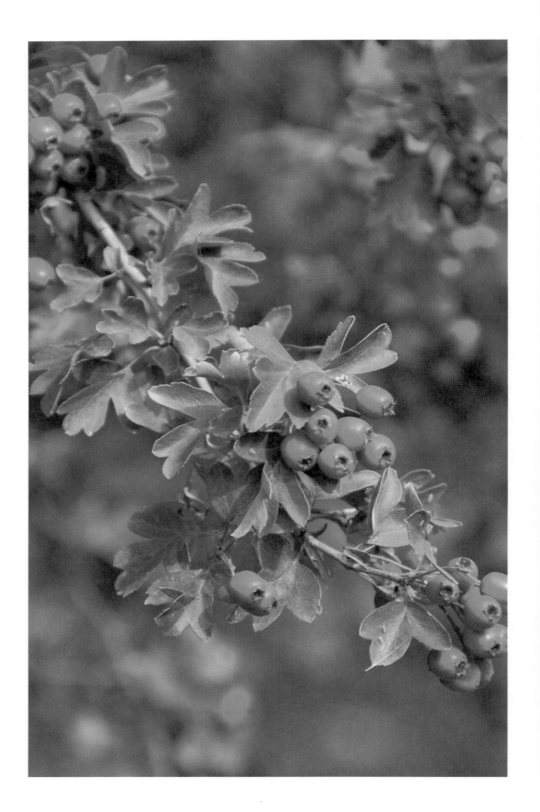

You will need

* 4.5 liters (1 gallon) water
* 1.8–2.7 kg (4–6 lb) Haws
* 225 g (8 oz) sultanas, chopped
* 5 ml (1 teaspoon) pectic enzyme powder
* 1 Campden tablet, crushed
* 1 lemon, thinly pared and squeezed
* 1.2 kg (2½ lb) sugar
* yeast and nutrient

Method

1 Bring the water to a boil and put the Haws in a fermenting bin with the sultanas. Pour the boiling water over the fruit and stir well. Cover and leave to cool.

2 When the water has cooled, crush the contents of the bin with a potato masher (or your choice of implement), then add the pectic enzyme and crushed Campden tablet, and the lemon zest and juice.

3 Cover and leave to infuse for two days, stirring often and crushing the Haws against the sides of the bin.

4 Pour in the sugar, stirring well to dissolve it, and add the yeast. Cover and leave in a warm place to ferment, stirring frequently and pressing down the cap that rises to the surface.

5 After about five days, strain off the liquid, squeezing gently to make sure you obtain it all, and transfer it to a demijohn. Fit the airlock and leave in a warm place to ferment, racking as required.

6 When fermentation has come to an end, siphon the wine off into a clean demijohn, fit the airlock, and store it in a cooler place for a week or two to allow it to settle.

7 A further sediment may form. When this is stable and the wine is completely clear, bottle, cork, and label. Store the wine for at least six months.

Lemon
Citrus limon

Like other citrus fruits, Lemons are thought to originate from Southeast Asia, from where they travelled west through trade. They had reached Persia well over two thousand years ago, and arrived in Europe in the Middle Ages. Citrus fruit are now grown commercially in California and the Mediterranean region. Bursting with citric acid, Lemon juice is traditionally used in western kitchens wherever a sharp taste is required. Most of the aromatic flavor comes from the rinds or zests, which is why these too are used so much in cooking. Lemon trees are small and spiny with waxy pale green leaves and deliciously fragrant white or purple flowers that belie the acid sharpness of the fruit. Grapefruit (*Citrus × paradisi*) is a Lemon hybrid which can be blended with Lemon to make a drinkable wine. (See pages 130–131 for a recipe.)

Loganberry
Rubus × loganobaccus

A cross between a blackberry and a raspberry, the first Loganberries were raised in California in the 1880s by an amateur horticulturist, Judge James Harvey Logan. They are said to have been produced by accident, when two varieties of blackberry being used in an experiment to breed a more reliable and earlier ripening form of the fruit hybridized with nearby raspberry plants.

In appearance, Loganberries are like elongated raspberries and they grow on canes much like raspberry canes but with the blackberry vigor, fruiting in late summer from inconspicuous flowers. In taste, the fruits are much sharper, but this makes them good for cooking and for use in preserves. The stems spread widely – up to 2.4 m (8 ft) – and grow to a height of 1.8 m (6 ft).

Loganberries are a garden plant, not normally found growing in the wild. They will grow in any ordinary, well-drained, well-composted soil in a sheltered position with some sun. It is best to train the stems on wires and to cut them down immediately after fruiting to encourage new ones to grow. Pick the fruits as they ripen and use them within a few days. With their fruity acidity, the berries make a pleasant, deep pink wine.

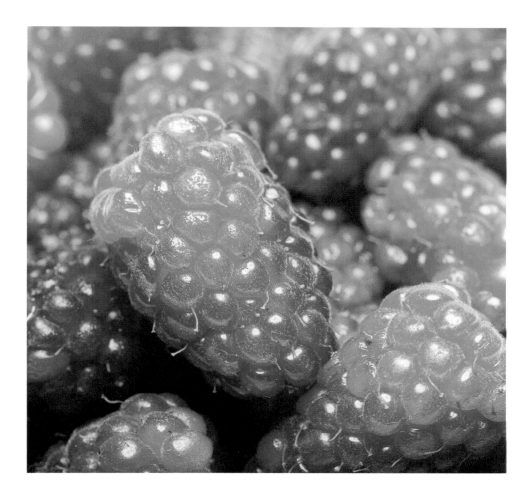

Loganberry Wine

This is a rosy-red wine with a light, fruity flavor. Pick just-ripe berries on a sunny day and either use them straight away or freeze them for later use. Inspect the berries for any obvious insects, then rinse them quickly before using or freezing.

You will need
* 1.3 kg (3 lb) Loganberries
* 1.3 kg (3 lb) sugar
* 4.5 liters (1 gallon) water
* yeast and nutrient (see Note, page 120)
* 2.5 ml (½ teaspoon) pectic enzyme powder

Method

1 Crush the fruit in a fermenting bin and add the sugar.
2 Boil the water and pour it into the bin, stirring to dissolve the sugar.
3 Cover and cool to 21–24°C (70–75°F). Add the yeast and pectic enzyme powder, stir, and cover.
4 Leave in a warm place to ferment for up to a week, stirring twice daily and pushing down the cap that comes to the surface.
5 Strain the liquid into a large container, squeezing the pulp gently to extract all the juice. Transfer to a demijohn and fit the airlock.
6 Ferment in a warm place, racking as needed.
7 When fermentation has stopped and the wine is clear, bottle, cork, and label. Store for a year.

Notes

* This wine improves with age, and can be served as Port.
* A Port yeast can be used instead of all-purpose yeast.

Medlar

Mespillus germanica

The Medlar tree comes mainly from coastal areas of present-day Turkey, where it has been cultivated for its fruits for thousands of years. The coastal situation provides the mild winters and hot summers that the plant thrives on. Some people believe it is also native to the British Isles, where it has certainly been grown for many centuries and can be found naturalized in some counties.

Though it can become an attractive gnarled and branching tree up to 7.5 m (25 ft) tall, it often makes a lower-growing shrubby plant with angled branches. The white flowers of mid-spring to early summer have five crumpled petals and are about 2.5–3.5 cm (1–1½ in) across. The downy, elliptic leaves are large in relation to the flowers – up to 15 cm (6 in) long and 4 cm (1¾ in) wide – and turn gold, then red, in the autumn before they fall.

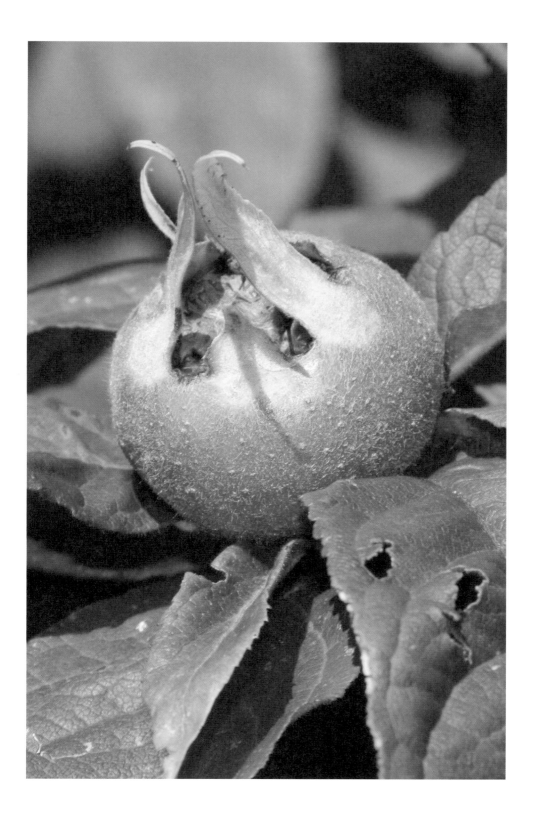

Medlar fruits are brownish in color, and related to apples and hawthorns. Firm and rounded, they have flat bottoms with a ring of distinctive sepals remaining from the outside of the flowers, and are extremely acidic. The hard fruits gradually soften up and become wrinkled on storage or if left on the tree until the frosts, until finally the fruit is soft, creamy, and edible – a process known as 'bletting.' Much cultivated in ancient Iran, by the Romans, and in medieval times, Medlars began to go out of fashion in the eighteenth century, but are getting to be better known again today.

You'll find them very occasionally on sale in country stores or direct from farms but anyone growing a Medlar is bound to have some fruit to spare.

Medlar Wine

First 'blet' your Medlars! Only Medlars that have been matured on the tree during the winter frosts, or stored on trays until they are wrinkled on the outsides, are soft and palatable enough to be used.

You will need
* 3.6 kg (8 lb) Medlars, crushed
* 225 g (8 oz) raisins, chopped
* 1 Campden tablet, crushed
* 4.5 liters (1 gallon) water
* 5 ml (1 teaspoon) peptic enzyme powder
* 1.2 kg (2½ lb) sugar
* yeast and nutrient

Method

1 Place the crushed Medlars in a fermenting bin, or crush them well in the bin. Add the chopped raisins and the crushed Campden tablet.

2 Bring the water to a boil and pour it into the bin. Stir, cover, and leave to steep for a week, adding the pectic enzyme powder when the liquid is cool and stirring twice daily. Activate the yeast toward the end of this time (see page 35).

3 Strain off the liquid, without pressing. Put it in a bin or large container, and stir in the sugar, making sure all the sugar dissolves. Add the yeast, stir, cover, and leave to ferment in a warm place for 24 hours, stirring twice.

4 Transfer to a demijohn, fit the airlock, and leave in a warm place to ferment. Rack as required as the sediment forms.

5 When the wine is clear and bubbling has ceased, siphon it into bottles, cork, and label. Store for six months.

Notes

* If you squeeze the straining bag in Step 3, there is a risk of cloudy wine. Instead, to extract the last drop of juice you can hang the bag over a bowl until the dripping stops.

* This makes a fairly sweet white wine, and Sauternes yeast may be used instead of all-purpose yeast.

Mulberry

Morus nigra

also known as Black Mulberry, Common Mulberry

The origins of the gnarled and stately Mulberry tree seem to be lost in time, and it has been cultivated for so long and in such widespread parts of the world that there are now very many different forms with experts in dispute about how to differentiate them.

No one disputes, however, that this long-lived tree makes a fine specimen for the garden lawn, and that its fruits are excellent, whether eaten fresh or made into tarts, jams, and jellies, while Mulberry Wine and syrup are rightly prized.

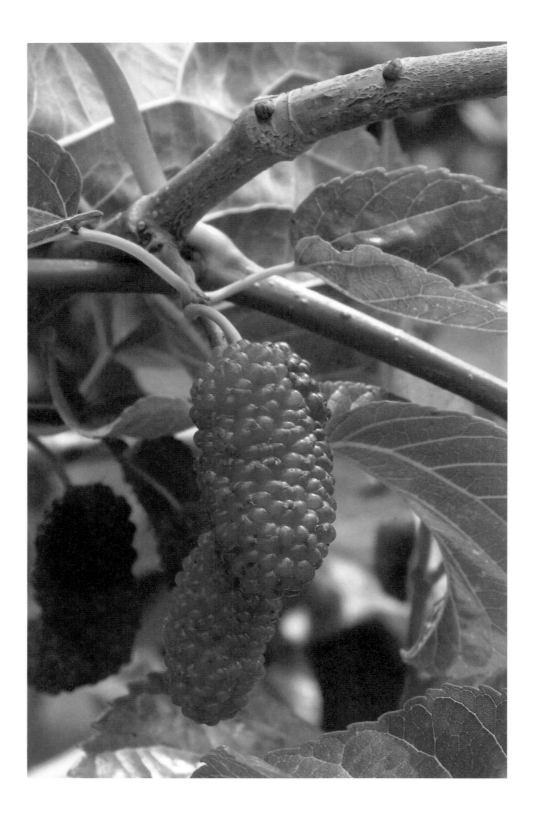

The Mulberry tree has bright, vine-like foliage in late spring and summer. This turns to golden yellow in the autumn and the Mulberry's spreading, twisting boughs can be appreciated in winter. The raspberry-like fruits grow from small, catkin-like flowers of no particular significance, but the fruits themselves are red to purple, turning black when fully ripe in late summer or early autumn, about 4 cm (1¾ in) in length, and very juicy. The trees grow slowly and can live to a great age, eventually with a height and spread of 6 m (20 ft), cropping generously year after year.

You'll find them Mulberries are not sold commercially as they have a short 'shelf life' and don't travel well. You may be lucky and find some on offer outside a country house with an old tree in its garden, or perhaps you have a friend who has a fruitful tree and wants to share its bounty.

Gathering the fruit If you have your own Mulberry tree, simply spread a large old sheet beneath it as the first fruits ripen and begin to fall. Gather up the sheet when you have the amount you need.

Tree for silkworms The sixteenth-century herbalist John Gerard describes the tree as follows: 'The common Mulberrie tree is high, and ful of boughes... Mulberrie trees grow plentifully in Italy and other hot regions, where they doe maintaine great woods and groves of them, that their Silke wormes may feed thereon.'

During the reign of James I, thousands of Black Mulberry trees were imported into Britain to foster the silk industry. In fact, however, the tree that fussy silkworms dined on proved to be the White Mulberry (*Morus alba*), so the operation was not a success. But Britain still has a number of very ancient trees whose pedigree dates back to the 1600s as a result of this experiment.

Caution The Black Mulberry is also cultivated in the United States, particularly in the south. It must not be confused with the native Red Mulberry, *Morus rubra*, a species which should be left alone, except by qualified medical herbalists, as its unripe fruit and the milky juices of its leaves are seriously hazardous to health.

Mulberry Wine

Use only really ripe Mulberries for this medium-dry red wine, picking them when they are black and ready to fall from the tree, or catching them in a cloth laid out on the ground. Unripe Mulberries are too acid and have not developed their full flavor. The juices develop as the fruits ripen.

You will need

* 2.7 kg (6 lb) Mulberries
* 225 g (8 oz) raisins, chopped
* 1.3 kg (3 lb) sugar
* 4.5 liters (1 gallon) water
* yeast and nutrient
* 2.5 ml (½ teaspoon) pectic enzyme powder

Method

1   Put the Mulberries in a fermenting bin and crush them against the sides to get the juices running.
2   Add the chopped raisins and stir in the sugar. Boil the water and pour it over the fruit, stirring well to dissolve the sugar.
3   Allow to cool to blood heat, then add the yeast and pectic enzyme powder.
4   Stir, cover, and leave to ferment for four days, stirring twice daily and pushing down the cap that rises to the top.
5   Strain through a fine strainer, squeezing gently to extract the juice.
6   Transfer to a demijohn, fit the airlock, and put in a warm place for fermenting to continue. Rack as necessary.
7   When fermenting has ceased and the wine is clear, move the demijohn to a cooler place for one week, then bottle, cork, and label. Store the wine for a year before serving.

Orange

Citrus × sinensis

also known as Sweet Orange

Oranges were cultivated in China more than two thousand years ago, and possibly originate from there (the name *sinensis* means 'from China'). Arab traders brought the bitter Orange to Europe at some time during the first millennium, and sweet Oranges were not known in the west until the fourteenth or even fifteenth centuries – nevertheless, long enough ago for them to be a household fruit and a long-time ingredient in our diets.

The familiar fruits grow on beautiful evergreen trees with scented, rather waxy, creamy white flowers that flourish in tropical, semi-tropical, and Mediterranean climates. Oranges are available in the shops year round and may come from Spain, North Africa, Brazil, California, Florida, Texas, or South Africa, depending on the season. Orange trees need temperatures of 16–29°C (60–84°F) to thrive and produce fruit. They are an important commercial crop in many parts of the world, and nowadays are often harvested mechanically using shaking machines. The fruits are green when unripe, ripening to the familiar orange color.

Orangery Growing Orange trees as ornamental plants was fashionable among the wealthy by the early eighteenth century, but the expensive plants were susceptible to cold weather, so that buildings were increasingly created to house them during the winter. In the stately homes of northern Europe, an elegant glazed orangery was *de rigueur*. An influential and very early example was the Orangerie at the Louvre Palace in Paris, built in 1617.

Orange Wine

Choose juicy, sweet Oranges to make this light, Sherry-like wine, and add a lemon for sharpness. Since the simplest way to make the wine is to juice the oranges, it is also a perfect way to use up spare cartons of Orange juice left over from a party.

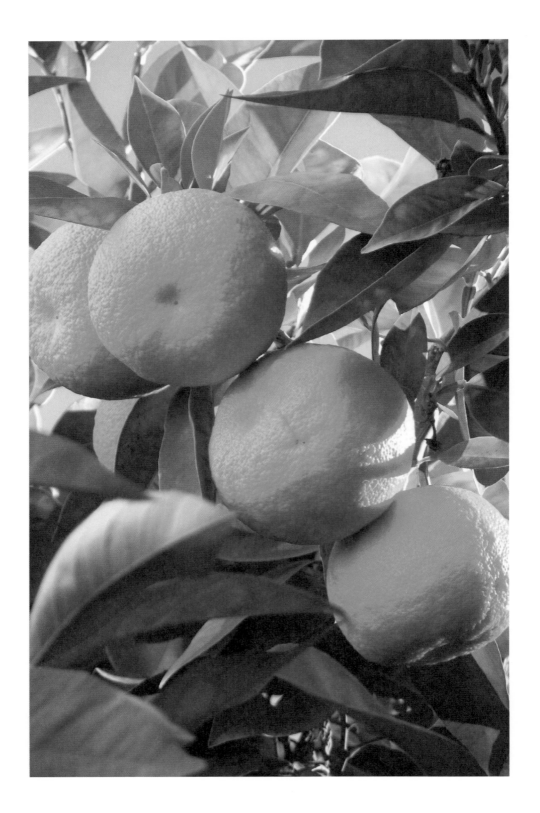

You will need

* 1 liter (2 pints) Orange juice, freshly squeezed or carton
* 175 g (6 oz) sultanas, chopped
* thinly pared zest of 4 Oranges (see Note below)
* 1 lemon, squeezed
* 1 Campden tablet, crushed
* 2.5 ml (½ teaspoon) grape tannin
* 3.5 liters (6 pints) water
* yeast and nutrient
* 1.3 kg (3 lb) sugar

Method

1   Put the Orange juice, sultanas, pared zest, lemon juice, crushed Campden tablet and grape tannin into a fermenting bin and add the water. Cover and leave to steep for 24 hours.
2   Stir the contents of the bin twice during the steeping time and activate the yeast towards the end of this period (see page 35).
3   Pour in all the sugar, and stir until it is completely dissolved, then add the yeast. Cover and leave to ferment in a warm place for four days, stirring twice daily.
4   Strain off the liquid into a demijohn, fit the airlock, and allow to ferment, racking as the sediment forms.
5   When fermentation has come to an end and the wine is clear, bottle, cork, and label. Store for at least six months.

Note

* Wash and scrub the skins of four of the Oranges and pare the zest very finely before you squeeze out the juice. Be careful not to include any pith as it will affect the taste of the wine.

Citrus Mix Wine

This makes a Grapefruit, Lemon, and Orange Wine with a fresh and fruity tang. The proportions of fruit can be varied to suit the situation. The fruits supply plenty of acid, so no acid blend is needed.

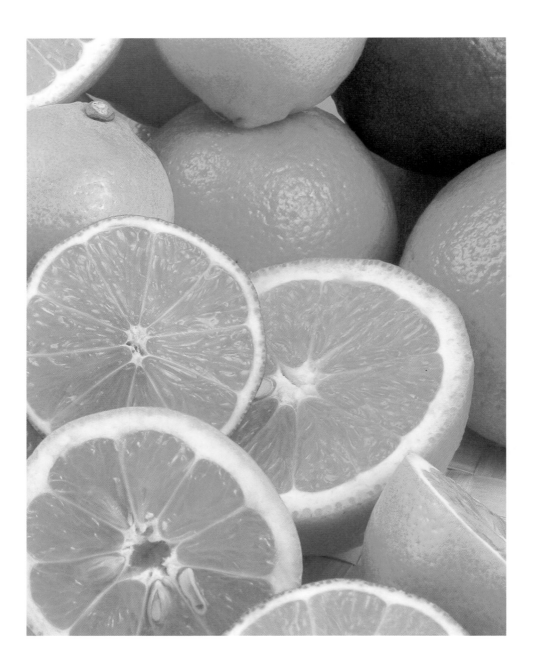

You will need

* 2 Grapefruits
* 2 Oranges
* 4 Lemons
* 100 g (4 oz) sultanas, chopped
* 2.5 ml (½ teaspoon) grape tannin
* 1.3 kg (3 lb) sugar
* up to 4.5 liters (1 gallon) water (see Method)
* 1 Campden tablet, crushed
* yeast and nutrient

Method

1 Wash and scrub the skins of the Grapefruits, the Oranges, and two of the Lemons, then thinly pare the zest. Put the parings into a fermenting bin and add the chopped sultanas and grape tannin.

2 Squeeze the juices from all the fruits into a measuring jug and note the quantity. Add the juices to the bin and stir in the sugar. Add the amount of water necessary to make the liquid up to 4.5 liters (1 gallon) and the crushed Campden tablet.

3 Stir to dissolve the sugar. Cover and steep for 24 hours, stirring twice. Activate the yeast towards the end of this period and follow the rest of the method as for Orange Wine (p 129).

Peach

Prunus persica

Like apricots (see page 79), Peaches originate from China. Prized by the ancient Chinese Emperors, they travelled west along the old Silk Route and were long ago introduced to Europeans. Flourishing in southern parts of North America and in the southern hemisphere, Peaches are also grown in Europe, but in England they need a warm, sunny wall, and those produced successfully in the past were often cosseted under glass.

Peach trees vary in height from 4 to 10 m (13–33 ft). The leaves are lance like, up to 15 cm (6 in) long, and the flowers appear in early spring before the leaves, singly or in pairs, about 2.5 cm (1 in) across, shell-pink, and delicately scented. Juicy and fleshy, the yellow or white fruits have crinkly stones with almond-like 'nuts' inside them. Unfortunately, the commercial crops often lack the qualities of the perfect Peach.

You'll find it This is not a fruit that many people will be lucky enough to gather or even buy from their local fruit farm, but the fruits are low in price toward the end of summer, and dried or canned Peaches can be used.

Colonial connection George Menifie (or Minifie), an early English settler in Virginia, is thought to have introduced Peaches to the New World in the 1630s, when he cultivated a large and beautiful garden with an orchard; their spread is believed to be due to indigenous people then planting the stones wherever they went. Peaches were grown by Thomas Jefferson at Monticello, his Virginian estate, and commercial production began in the nineteenth century.

Peach Wine

Peaches make a sweet, fruity-flavored white wine for dessert in this recipe, but drier versions can be made and any recipe for Apricot Wine would be suitable for Peaches. Yellow-fleshed, freestone varieties – not white or cling Peaches – are the ones to use.

You will need
* 1.8 kg (4 lb) ripe fresh Peaches (450 g/1 lb dry)
* 10 ml (2 teaspoons) acid blend
* 2.5 ml (½ teaspoon) grape tannin
* 4.5 liters (1 gallon) water
* 1.3 kg (3 lb) sugar
* 2.5 ml (½ teaspoon) pectic enzyme powder
* yeast and nutrient
* finings (optional, see Method)
* 1 vitamin C tablet, crushed

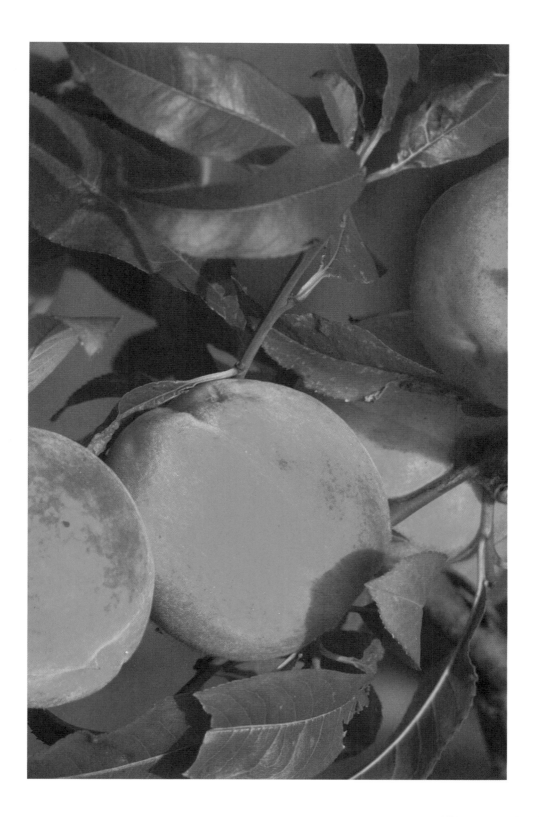

Method

1 Remove the stones from the Peaches, cut up the Peaches and crush the fruit in a fermenting bin. Add the acid blend and grape tannin. Keep covered while you bring the water to a boil.

2 Stir in the sugar and pour on the hot water. Stir to make sure that the sugar is completely dissolved, cover, and leave to cool.

3 When the pulp is at 21–24°C (70–75°F), add the pectic enzyme powder and the yeast, cover again, and leave to ferment for about six days, stirring well twice daily.

4 Strain off the liquid, pressing gently to get all the juice, then transfer it to a demijohn and fit the airlock. Leave the wine to ferment in a warm place.

5 Rack as necessary as the wine clears and a sediment forms. Finings can be used if the wine seems very slow to clear (following the packet instructions).

6 When the wine is clear and fermentation has stopped, add a crushed vitamin C tablet to prevent discoloration. Bottle, cork, and label. Store for a year.

Pear

Pyrus communis
also known as Common Pear

The Common Pear grows wild in Europe except in the far north and south, and as with apples the fruits of the wild trees are small, hard, and sour, unless they are from trees that have escaped into the countryside from orchards and gardens. Pears may have originated in the mountains of central Asia and probably spread and hybridized of their own accord, rather than by trade.

The parent of modern cultivated varieties of Pear is native to an area from western Europe to the Himalayas, but generally Pears do not like more northern parts. The trees are pyramidal in shape and up to 20 m (65 ft) high, with attractive white blossom in early or mid-spring. The fruit itself is too well known to need description. Most Pears do not store well and have always been used for making drinks. Wine from the juice of pears is known as Perry.

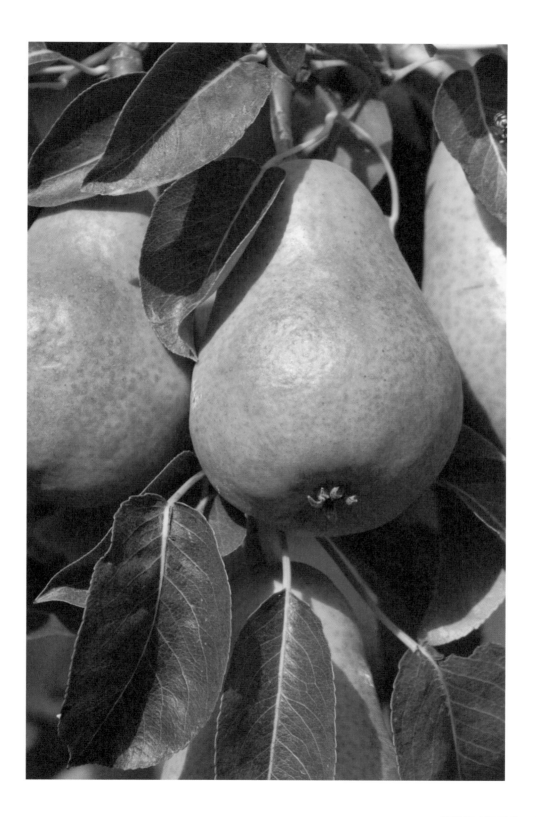

Many an old garden has an over-productive Pear tree or two. They flourish best in warmth, sun, and shelter, though they are tolerant of wet conditions and always require some moisture in the soil. Pears cannot stand cold winds and even the self-fertile varieties generally do better with partners.

You'll find it   Wild Pears may be found growing alone in light woodland, in hedgerows, and at field margins, sometimes marking the site of an old orchard.

Digestive drink   The herbalist John Gerard (1545–1612) mentions wild Pears and their wine: 'Wine made of the juice of pears is called in English, Perry [it] purgeth those that are not accustomed to drinke thereof, especially when it is new; notwithstanding it is as wholesome a drinke being taken in small quantities as wine; it comforteth and warmeth the stomacke, and causeth good digestion.'

Pear Wine

Pear Wine has a reputation for being a tricky one to make. Pears are generally low in acid, so need a boost from acid blend or lemon juice, and the wine clouds easily, so the pectic enzyme is essential. A mix of ripe and unripe Pears is best.

You will need
* 2.7 kg (6 lb) Pears, wiped clean
* 4.5 liters (1 gallon) water
* 2 Campden tablets, crushed
* 2.5 ml (½ teaspoon) pectic enzyme powder
* yeast and nutrient
* 1.2 kg (2½) lb sugar
* 20 ml (4 teaspoons) acid blend
* 1 vitamin C tablet, crushed
* finings (see Method)

Method

1 Chop or crush the Pears and put them in a fermenting bin or large container.
2 Heat the water to boiling point, and pour it over the Pears. Add a crushed Campden tablet.
3 Cover and steep for three days, adding in the pectic enzyme powder when the liquid has cooled. Stir daily.
4 Activate the yeast at the end of this period (see page 35).
5 Strain off the liquid, pressing the solids very gently to get all the juices, then pour it over the sugar in a fermenting bin. Stir well, making sure that the sugar is fully dissolved.
6 Add the acid blend and yeast, cover, and leave to ferment for four or five days, stirring daily.
7 Siphon the liquid into a demijohn, fit the airlock, and leave to ferment, racking as required.
8 When the wine is clear and fermentation has ceased,, siphon into a clean jar. Add the vitamin C tablet and a crushed Campden tablet to prevent browning. Fit a bung and move it to a cooler place to mature.
9 After two months, siphon off into bottles, cork, and label. Store for a year.

Notes

* Pear Wine can be cloudy and slow to clear, so may need to be cleared with finings, following the instructions on the packet.
* The juice of two lemons can be used instead of the acid blend. True wild Pears are much more acid, and little further acid will be needed in this case.

Plum
see page 95

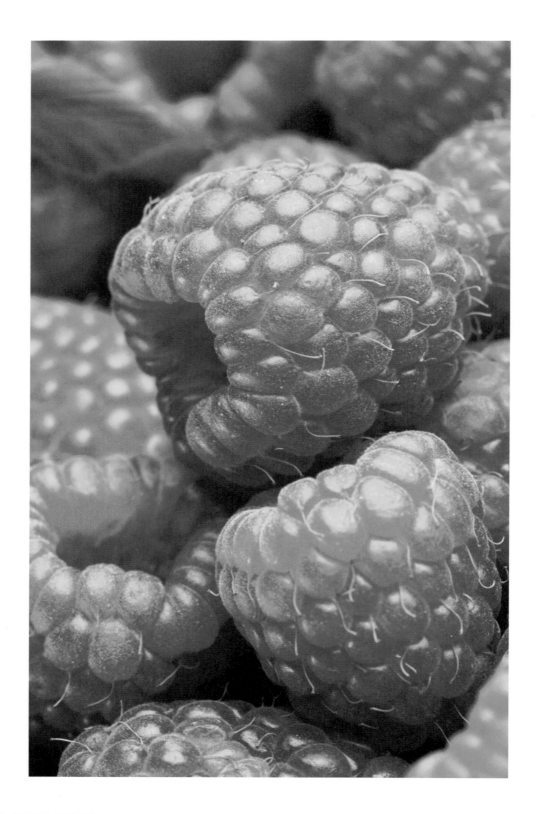

Raspberry

Rubus idaeus

also known as European Raspberry, Framboise, Hindberry, Rasps

Raspberry plants grow wild in many parts of Europe, Asia, and North America, and are native to all these areas, though often the plants growing in the wild today will have escaped from gardens. The unbranched stems (known as canes) bend as they lengthen and grow to a length of up to 1.5 m (5 ft). The canes are gently prickly and the leaves have three or five tooth-edged leaflets, grey on the backs and slightly rough. Each year's fruits are borne on canes thrown up the previous summer. The small flowers that appear from early summer are pinkish-white, and develop into the well-known summer fruit. In the wild, the fruits are usually smaller than cultivated Raspberries, but with an intense flavor. Cultivated Raspberries are fairly easy to grow in the garden, if you can give them a loamy soil that holds its moisture, and are available for sale in shops throughout the summer and into early autumn, as well as in pick-your-own fruit farms.

You'll find it in light woods, in hedgerows, and on heaths and hillsides. Sometimes the plants grow prolifically but more often they are shy, so it is best not to pick wild Raspberries unless they are particularly plentiful.

Raspberry Wine

Raspberries make a lovely rosé or light red wine, which can be dry or sweet, depending on your preference. Use berries that are sound and ripe and wash them quickly in a colander to make sure they are free of insects.

You will need
* 1.3 kg (3 lb) Raspberries
* 2.5 ml (½ teaspoon) grape tannin
* 2.5 ml (½ teaspoon) acid blend
* 1 Campden tablet, crushed
* 5 ml (1 teaspoon) pectic enzyme powder
* 1.2 kg (2½ lb) sugar (or 1.3 kg/3 lb for a sweeter wine)
* 4.5 liters (1 gallon) water
* yeast and nutrient

Method

1 Crush the fruit in a fermenting bin. Mix in the grape tannin, acid blend, crushed Campden tablet, and pectic enzyme powder.

2 Add the sugar, bring the water to a boil, and pour it over the fruit. Stir to dissolve all the sugar. Cover and stand for 24 hours.

3 Add the yeast to the bin, cover, and leave to ferment for six days, stirring daily.

4 Strain the liquid from the solids, extracting all the juice. Transfer it into a demijohn, fit the fermentation lock, and stand in a warm place. Rack as required as fermentation continues (usually after three weeks and again after three months).

5 Bottle when fermentation has come to an end and the wine is clear. Cork and label. Store for one year.

Redcurrant

Ribes rubrum

also known as Northern Redcurrant, Wineberry

Redcurrant and Blackcurrant (see page 87) plants are very similar, but differ in that the Redcurrant is a shapely bush that generally has one main stem with branches growing from it, while Blackcurrant bushes have multiple stems. Redcurrant leaves are five-lobed and clusters of small, greenish flowers grow from the leaf joints in mid- to late spring, followed in mid-summer by hanging strings (known as 'strigs') of clear red, almost transparent berries. The fruit is sharp and acid, but with a distinctive and sought-after flavor.

These shrubs are widely native in western Europe, spreading into Scandinavia, Russia, and Asia. They are also found growing wild in North America and are cultivated in many countries. They grow mainly in a cool climate, but like a sunny position with protection from wind.

Unless wild fruits are very plentiful, it is best to grow your own, or buy them when they are in season. Many pick-your-own farms produce Redcurrants, which are especially in demand for jams and jellies. The season is quite brief, so make the most of it.

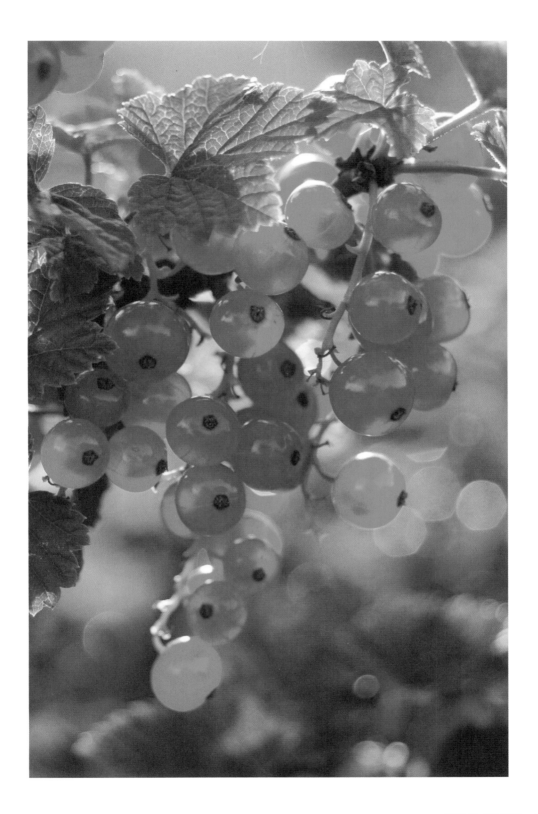

You'll find it in hedgerows and light woodland in well-drained but moisture-retentive soils, and more frequently in mountain woods or damp and rocky moorland places.

Redcurrant Wine

This recipe makes a clear rosé wine that is relatively dry for a country wine, bringing out some of the sharpness in the Redcurrant flavor. Freezing the fruit will help to break down the pectin and maximize the juice yield.

You will need

* 1.3 kg (3 lb) Redcurrants, fresh or frozen
* 4.5 liters (1 gallon) boiling water
* 1 Campden tablet, crushed
* 5 ml (1 teaspoon) pectic enzyme powder
* yeast and nutrient
* 1.2 kg (2½ lb) sugar

Method

1 Put the prepared Redcurrants into a fermenting bin, crush them with a wooden spoon or rolling pin, and pour the boiling water over them (see Note opposite).

2 Cover and leave to cool, then stir in the crushed Campden tablet and the pectic enzyme powder. Cover again and leave to steep for 24 hours, stirring once or twice.

3 Activate the yeast (see page 35) and stir the sugar into the Redcurrant infusion, making sure that it is well dissolved. Add the activated yeast, cover, and ferment for about five days, stirring and pushing down the cap once or twice a day.

4 Strain off the liquid and transfer it to a demijohn. Fit the airlock and ferment in a warm place, racking as required.

5 When fermentation has stopped, siphon the wine into dark bottles to protect it from the light. Cork and label. Store for a minimum of one year.

Notes

* Redcurrants are high in pectin, so the pectic enzyme is essential, especially when fresh berries are used.
* You may prefer to put the fruit into a jumbo straining bag in Step 1, before crushing.

Rosehip
Rosa canina
also known as Briar Rose, Dog Rose, Wild Rose

To most country lovers the Wild Rose needs no introduction. Swathed over the hedgerows in early summer, or forming beautiful shrubs in its own right, its pale pink, lightly rose-scented flowers are a sure sign of summer being almost here. The wide-open flowers are five-petalled and delicate with golden stamens in the centers. White forms are also often found. The stems on which they grow are long (to 3–4 m/10–13 ft) and arching and well supplied with sharp spines. The slightly prickly leaves consist of two or three pairs of tooth-edged leaflets with one extra topping them off.

The flowers of Wild Roses develop into bright red, urn-shaped or egg-shaped hips at the end of summer. The hips are yellowish inside with mealy flesh that is packed with hairy, hard seeds; they last long on the bushes and are very popular with birds. When gathering Rosehips, take care to leave plenty to provide the birds with winter pickings.

You'll find it Wild Rosehips are widely found in temperate parts of the northern hemisphere, with different regions having their own related species of Rose. They grow in hedgerows and on grazing land, on hillsides, and beside country paths.

Nature's bounty We all know that oranges are rich in vitamin C, and most people think of blackcurrants as another excellent source of this vital vitamin. But the hips of the Wild Rose in fact contain more vitamin C than any other fruit – or vegetable. Weight for weight, they supply 20 times the amount that is found in oranges.

Rosehip Wine

Wild Rosehips make a fairly dry white wine. A food mincer is useful for preparing the hips, which should be picked after the frosts have softened them and made them a little less sour. There are many country recipes and variations.

You will need

* 1.8–2.3 kg (4–5 lb) fresh Rosehips or 175–225 g (6–8 oz) dried
* 225 g (8 oz) raisins (optional, see Note opposite)
* 1.3 kg (3 lb) sugar (see Note opposite)
* 2 oranges, pared and squeezed
* 2 lemons, pared and squeezed
* 4.5 liters (1 gallon) boiling water
* yeast and nutrient
* 1 Campden tablet, crushed
* 1 vitamin C tablet, crushed

Method

1   Mince the Rosehips or cut them in half. Mix in a fermenting bin with the raisins, sugar, zest and juice of the oranges and lemons, and boiling water. Stir well to dissolve the sugar.
2   Cover and leave to cool. When the contents of the bin have cooled to 21°C (70°F), add the yeast and nutrient.
3   Cover and leave to ferment for five days, stirring twice daily, pressing the Rosehips against the sides and pushing down the cap that rises to the surface.
4   Carefully strain the fermenting juices off the solids, using a very fine straining cloth. Strain again to make quite sure that there are no hairs left in the liquid.
5   Siphon (or pour) the liquid into a demijohn, fit the airlock and leave in a warm place to ferment, racking as the contents clear and sediment forms (see Note opposite).
6   When there is no more activity and the wine is clear, siphon into a clean jar, add a crushed Campden tablet and a vitamin C tablet to keep the color pure, bung up the jar, and leave in a cool place for two more weeks.
7   Rack again if necessary, then bottle, cork, and label. Store for six months.

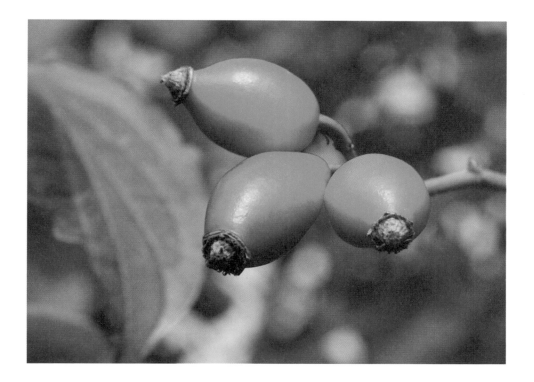

Notes

* If you wish to use raisins for a slightly fruitier taste, reduce the amount of sugar to 1.2 kg (2½) lb .

* Fermentation can be very rapid with Rosehip Wine. Be prepared to rack after the first three weeks and again two months later.

Sloe

Prunus spinosa

Sloes are the fruits of the Blackthorn, a widespread spiny shrub or small tree, 3–4.5 m (10–15 ft) high, stiff-growing, and with blackish stems and twigs. Blackthorns flower early in the spring, with clouds of airy, white blossom almost covering the dark branches. Small, matt, oval leaves follow, and the fruits appear in late summer to ripen in the autumn. Only about 12 mm (½ in) across, round and plum-like, dark inky blue in color but with a light blue bloom, the Sloes often outstay the yellowing leaves. The fruits are incredibly tart and inedible, raw or cooked, but as well as featuring in country jams and jellies they produce a really classic wine.

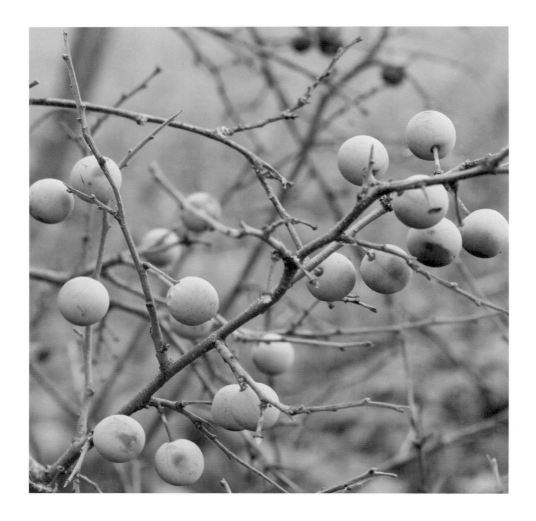

Native to Europe, Blackthorn has been introduced to North America, having been grown as a useful hedgerow plant on farmland. Blackthorn needs an open, sunny situation, but grows in almost any kind of soil, often forming thickets.

You'll find it in hedgerows, light woodland, scrubland, and farmland. Gather the fruits in mid- to late autumn, when they are fully ripe.

Sloe Wine

This recipe makes a slow-maturing, deep red wine. Sloe Wine may be less famous than the more alcoholic Sloe Gin, but is well worth making – either as a table wine, or, with the addition of vine fruits and a little more sugar, as a dessert wine.

You will need

* 1.3 kg (3 lb) ripe Sloes
* 4.5 liters (1 gallon) water
* 1 Campden tablet, crushed
* 5 ml (1 teaspoon) pectic enzyme
* 1.25 kg (2¾ lb) sugar
* yeast and nutrient

Method

1　Wash the Sloes, remove them from their stems and put them into a fermenting bin or large container.
2　Bring the water to a boil and pour it over the Sloes, stirring well. Cover and allow to cool, when the Sloes will be softened.
3　Crush the Sloes against the sides of the container, and stir in the crushed Campden tablet and the pectic enzyme. Cover and leave to infuse for four days.
4　Strain the infusion into a fermenting bin, pressing to extract all the juice, pour in the sugar, stir to dissolve the sugar completely, then add the yeast.
5　Cover and leave to ferment in a warm place for several days, stirring twice daily and pushing down the cap that rises.
6　Siphon into a demijohn, fit the airlock, and leave in a warm place to ferment, racking as required.
7　When fermentation has stopped and the wine is clear, transfer it to a clean demijohn, insert a bung, and leave for a year to mature in a cool, dark place.
8　Bottle, cork, and label at the end of this time. Store for at least a further year. The wine will repay a three-year wait.

Note

* For a dessert wine, add 225 g (8 oz) chopped raisins or sultanas (or a mix of both) in Step 1 and increase the amount of sugar used to 1.3 kg (3 lb), adding the extra in stages.

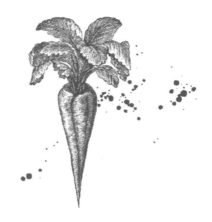

VEGETABLE
AND ROOT WINES

The vegetables for wines will not normally be found growing wild, but many are relatively easy to grow in a small garden, and making wines is a good way to use up surplus or over-mature produce. Many vegetables are particularly rich in starches to provide some sweetness, and in mucilaginous material which gives the yeast nitrogenous matter to feed on, but they are often lacking in acid, which must be boosted. A good deal of the flavor lies in the skins, so vegetables should never be peeled, though they should be washed and any damaged parts cut out.

Cutting vegetables into small pieces enables the maximum flavor to be extracted from them. Often the best way to extract the juices and flavors is to cook the chopped vegetables to softness and strain off the cooking liquor, which makes for very simple winemaking. The vegetables themselves need not be wasted and can be used afterwards for soups or purées. Older vegetables have stronger flavors and are better for wine than younger, more tender ones.

Beetroot
Beta vulgaris
also known as Beets

Ever popular, Beetroot is not a demanding vegetable to grow. It was introduced to Britain in late Tudor times and was said to come from southern Europe. Being a maritime plant, Beetroot enjoys some salt in its diet and thrives in gardens near the sea. It should be sown in mid- to late spring, depending on the kindness of the local climate, and given a well-drained or sandy soil if possible. The sweetness of the roots depends on the soil being kept moist.

Harvest Beets throughout the summer, and into early autumn. Pull them up by gripping the stalks and turning them, or ease them out of the ground gently with a fork, taking care not to damage them and make them 'bleed.' They are shallow rooted, so should come away easily. Twist off the leaves by hand rather than cutting with a knife, again to prevent 'bleeding.' (Incidentally, the leaves can be used to make the most delicious soup.) Use large, mature Beets for making country wine, which is one of the best vegetable wines, the sweetness and the color both contributing roundly to the beverage.

Master Lete's Beets
John Gerard, the English herbalist whose London garden was famous for the rare and interesting plants he grew, wrote of Beetroot in his *The Herbal, or a general histoire of plants* (1597), extolling the vegetable. It seems the plant he grew was 'the Great Red Beet' and that it was given to him by Master Lete, a London merchant and fellow plant collector.

Beetroot Wine
A well-made Beetroot Wine is a good rich red in color, but to achieve this it needs to be kept away from the light, during both fermenting and storing. The wine is slow to mature and repays a long wait with a true country flavor.

You will need

* 2.3 kg (5 lb) Beetroot
* 2 lemons
* 12 g (½ oz) root ginger, sliced
* 4.5 liters (1 gallon) water
* 1.3 kg (3 lb) sugar
* 2 oranges
* yeast and nutrient

Method

1 Wash and scrub the Beets, then slice them into a preserving pan or large saucepan. Pare the lemons and add the zest to the pan with the sliced ginger. Pour on the water, bring to a boil and simmer until the Beetroot is just tender.

2 Strain into a fermenting bin, stir in the sugar, allowing it to dissolve completely, and then squeeze in the juice of the lemons and oranges. Allow to cool to blood heat.

3 Add the yeast and nutrient, cover, and leave to ferment for about five days, stirring daily.

4 Siphon into a dark glass demijohn, fit the airlock, and keep in a warm place for fermentation to continue, racking as required.

5 When the wine is completely clear, and fermentation has stopped, bottle in dark bottles, cork, and label. Store for two years, away from light, to allow it to mature. (Alternatively, store the finished wine for a year in a dark jar or demijohn with a closely fitting stopper or bung, before bottling and storing for a further year.)

Notes

* If a dark demijohn is not available, fix brown wrapping paper to the jar to exclude the light.
* The cooked Beetroot can be used for soup or as a table vegetable.
* Use end-of-season Beets in preference to young ones.

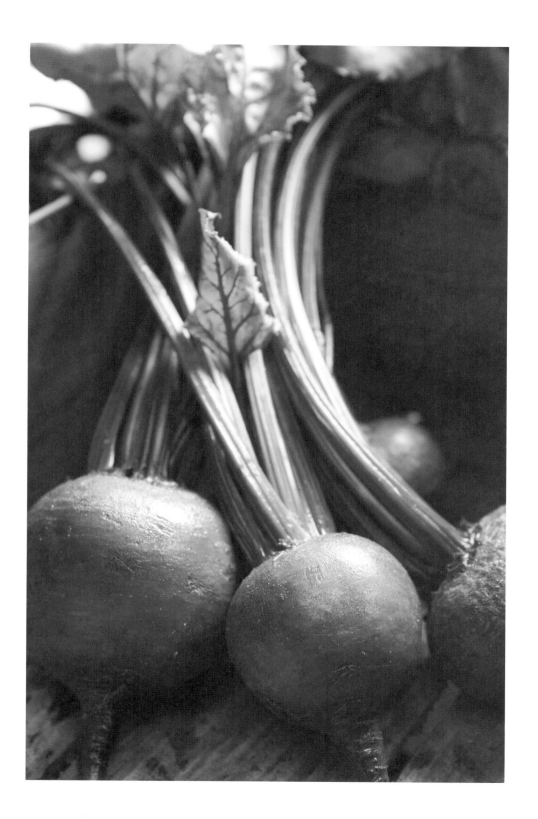

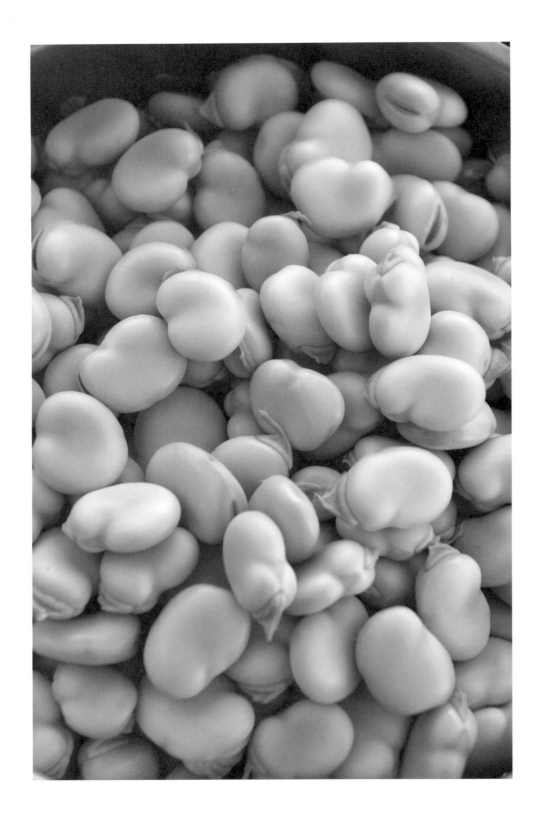

Broad Bean
Vicia faba
also known as Fava Beans

Broad Bean plants can yield prolific quantities of pods for a time, and it is not always possible to pick them all at their tender best. Luckily the slightly tough old beans you may get towards the end of the season are perfect for making wine. If you have a surplus, or are given beans by a neighbor and consider them a little past their best, you will find they make a good dry, light wine.

If you are thinking of growing Broad Beans yourself, you should dig and manure the ground in the autumn before sowing the seeds in late autumn (in mild areas only) or in early spring. You will need to give most varieties some means of support, and pinch out the first flowering tips to keep off blackfly. Other than this, they are rewarding and undemanding, and the ones you grow are so much better than the ones on sale – except perhaps from local market gardens or outside someone's house on weekend walks. Harvest by pulling the whole pod from the main stems, then open the pod along the 'seam' to extract the beans. Broad Beans are quite starchy and you must take care not to let them split during boiling as this enables too much starch to be released, which causes hazy wine.

Broad Bean Wine

This recipe makes a clear white wine, which is a little reminiscent of a German table wine. Only the beans themselves are needed (and not the pods), but this is a very good way of using beans that are too old and large to be served as a vegetable.

You will need
* 1.8 kg (4 lb) Broad Beans, shelled
* 4.5 liters (1 gallon) water
* 1 lemon, pared and squeezed
* 100 g (4 oz) raisins, chopped
* 1.25 kg (2¾ lb) sugar
* 2.5 ml (½ teaspoon) grape tannin
* 5 ml (1 teaspoon) starch enzyme
* yeast and nutrient (see Note on page 154)
* finings (see Method)

Method

1   Bring the Broad Beans to a boil in the water, add the pared lemon zest and chopped raisins and simmer very gently for an hour.
2   Strain off the liquid into a fermenting bin and stir in the sugar, making sure that it dissolves completely. Cover and allow to cool to blood heat, then add the lemon juice, tannin, starch enzyme, and yeast.
3   Cover and leave to ferment for four days or until vigorous fermentation slows down, stirring frequently.
4   Siphon into a demijohn, fit the airlock, and leave in a warm place for fermentation to continue. Rack as the sediment forms.
5   When all activity has ceased, rack again. If the wine is still cloudy, finings may be needed to clear it (used according to the instructions on the packet).
6   Bottle, cork, and label. Store for six months to a year.

Note

∗ A Hock yeast can be used for this wine.

Carrot

Daucus carota

Another well-known vegetable, often cheap and plentiful in the shops, the humble Carrot is not to be despised by country winemakers. While early thinnings make a lovely vegetable or salad ingredient, large, old, end-of-season Carrots are sometimes uninviting vegetables for the table. Yet they contain much sweetness, and are perfect for making a wine that is reminiscent of Sherry.

Wild Carrots will not be found for winemaking, but this is a vegetable you may wish to grow, if you have well-drained, warm soil. Sow in early spring for a main crop, and never apply manure at the time of sowing or during the growing season. Pull the Carrots up by hand as you require them, but save some of the biggest of the crop for brewing. If you cannot get hold of homegrown Carrots you will find that the ones available in the shops are perfectly suitable too.

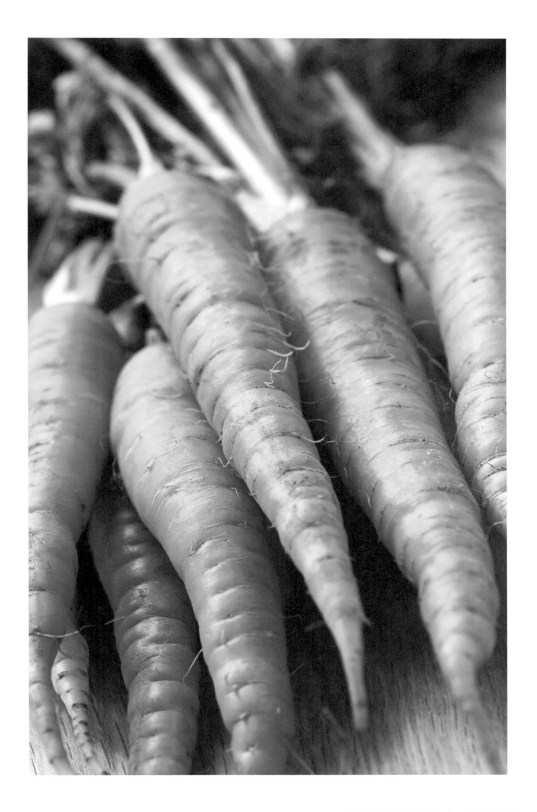

Cultivated Carrots Wild Carrots are native to large parts of the world, ranging from Europe to southwest Asia. The cultivated forms were probably introduced to Europe over a thousand years ago from the region of modern-day Iran and Afghanistan, and the specimens grown today came via the Netherlands during the seventeenth century.

Carrot Wine

Carrot Wine is thought to resemble Sherry, and a Sherry yeast can be used to replace all-purpose wine yeast in this recipe. The recipe makes a medium-sweet wine, which improves with age, so store it for at least a year before drinking.

You will need
* 1.8 kg (4 lb) Carrots
* 1 lemon, squeezed and thinly pared
* 1 orange, squeezed and thinly pared
* 4.5 liters (1 gallon) water
* 175 g (6 oz) raisins, chopped
* 1.2 kg (2½ lb) sugar
* 5 ml (1 teaspoon) grape tannin
* yeast and nutrient

Method
1 Wash, scrub, and slice the Carrots. Put them into a preserving pan or large saucepan with the pared zest. Bring to a boil in the water and simmer for 15 minutes or until the Carrots are tender.
2 Transfer to a fermenting bin, add the chopped raisins, sugar, and lemon and orange juice. Stir well to dissolve the sugar, and allow to cool to blood heat.
3 Add the tannin, yeast, and nutrient, cover and leave to ferment for about five days, stirring daily.
4 Strain, then siphon the liquid into a demijohn, fit the airlock, and keep in a warm place for fermentation to continue, racking as required.
5 When the wine is completely clear and fermentation has stopped, bottle, cork, and label it. Store the wine for two years, if possible, to allow it to mature fully.

Mangel Wurzel

Beta vulgaris **subsp.** *vulgaris*

Properly known as Mangel Beet or Mangold, the Mangel Wurzel likes to stick to its old country name. This sugar-rich root vegetable is closely related to Chard and Sugar Beet, and was developed as a fodder crop for cattle during the Agrarian Revolution of the eighteenth century. Its origins probably lie in a wild sea beet indigenous to southern and western Europe. Country folk soon developed two much more folkloric uses for the weighty yellow or white swollen roots, and saw that the Mangel Wurzel was perfect for winemaking and the village sport of hurling (see below). Many farmers grow Mangel Wurzels as a winter feed for their livestock. If you are not a farmer yourself, and don't grow them in your garden, you could try begging a few from a friendly farmer.

Hurling Hurling with vegetables has its roots in medieval times, and early in the nineteenth century the lads of the Somerset Levels in England developed the sport using hefty Mangel Wurzels, which were grasped by the stems and hurled towards the winning vegetable from the previous year. Since the Levels are prone to flooding, the hurler pitched his root while standing in a special woven pitching basket. Willow boys cut young stems from the local willow trees as rods for measuring the throw, and the Wurzel that was nearest to the mark became this year's prize-winner, the 'Norman.'

Mangel Wurzel Wine

This wine is fairly dry for a country wine, and can be served with food as a table wine. It is traditionally made in early spring, probably because the roots are then less starchy, and, as the farm animals are going out to graze, there is often a surplus.

You will need
* 2 kg (4½ lb) Mangel Wurzels
* 2 lemons
* 1 orange
* 4.5 liters (1 gallon) water
* 1.3 kg (3 lb) sugar
* 30 ml (2 tablespoons) strong cold tea
* yeast and nutrient

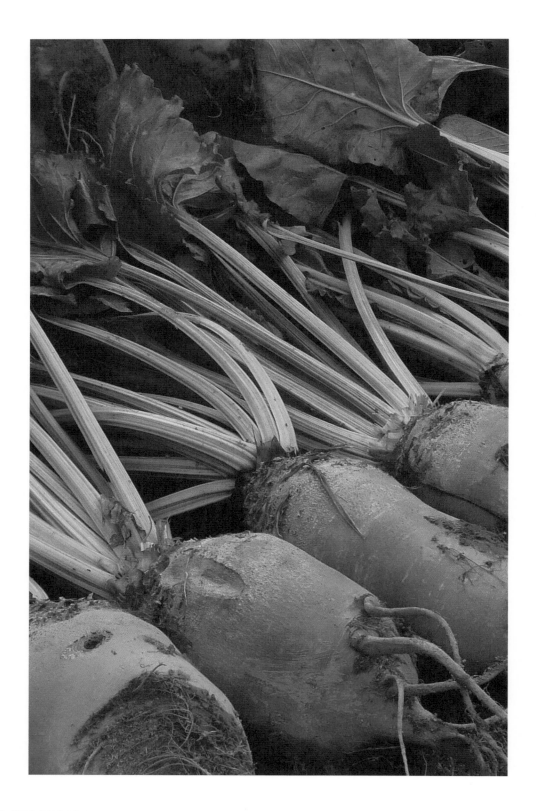

Method

1   Scrub the Wurzels and the citrus fruit. Dice the Wurzels, thinly pare the fruit, and put them together in a preserving pan or large saucepan. Bring to a boil in the water and simmer until the Wurzels are tender.

2   Strain into a fermenting bin, stir in the sugar, making sure that it dissolves completely, and add the juice of the lemons and orange with the cold tea. Allow to cool to blood heat.

3   Add the yeast and nutrient, cover, and leave to ferment for about a week, stirring daily.

4   Siphon into a demijohn, fit the airlock, and keep in a warm place for fermentation to continue, racking as required.

5   When the wine is clear, and fermentation has stopped, bottle, cork, and label. Store for at least nine months before drinking.

Notes

*   The wine may clear slowly – patience is required.
*   One medium-sized root will be about the right weight.

Marrow or Bush Marrow
Cucurbita pepo
also known as Summer Squash, Vegetable Marrow

Marrows arrived on our tables in the nineteenth century – relatively recently in terms of the food we grow – but they have become a classic late summer and autumn vegetable. Anyone who grows Marrows is bound to have a few to spare during the season. Like Carrots, they are best for the table when still young and tender. But there is no need to reject hard-skinned, heavy, mature specimens when it comes to making wine. While the big pips are found unwelcome by the cook, every part of the fruit (for Marrows are really fruits though treated as a vegetable) is used to make Marrow wine – a well-established country kitchen favorite. Cylindrical, striped dark green and cream, and often ridged, Marrows grow quickly in warm areas, requiring heat of 18–27°C (64–80°F) and doing best in soil that is well prepared with rotted compost or manure. Marrows are about 95 per cent water, and during dry weather they need to be kept watered. Harvest the fruit by cutting through the stem with a sharp knife while taking the Marrow's weight in the other hand.

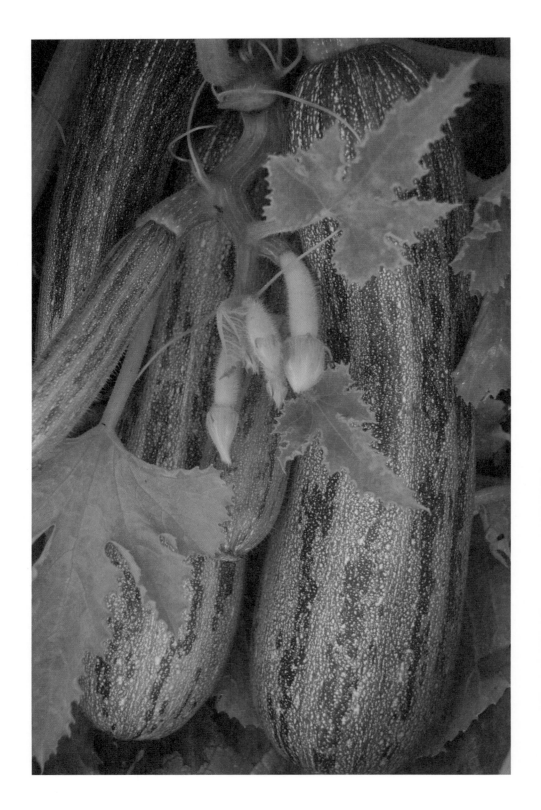

Marrow Wine (Squash Wine)

You might expect a wine made with what is rather a watery vegetable to be somewhat bland, but this version is enlivened with root ginger and enriched with Demerara sugar, which enhances the flavor and gives the wine a golden hue.

You will need

* 1 large marrow (weight about 2.7 kg/6 lb)
* 50 g (2 oz) piece of root ginger, sliced
* 100 g (4 oz) raisins, chopped
* 4.5 liters (1 gallon) water
* 1 Campden tablet, crushed
* 3 lemons
* 1.3 kg (3 lb) sugar
* yeast and nutrient

Method

1 Scrub the Marrow and leave it unpeeled. Cut or chop it into small pieces – skin, pips, core, and all – and put them into a fermenting bin with the sliced ginger and chopped raisins.
2 Boil the water and pour it into the bin. Give a good stir and add the crushed Campden tablet.
3 Cover and leave to steep for three days, stirring twice daily and pushing the Marrow pulp against the sides of the bin.
4 Squeeze the lemons and add the juice to the pulp. Stir in the sugar, stirring until it is dissolved, then sprinkle on the yeast.
5 Cover and keep in a warm place to ferment for a further three or four days, stirring as before and pushing down the cap that rises to the surface.
6 Strain through a very fine strainer and transfer the liquid to a demijohn, fit the airlock, and keep in a warm place while fermentation continues.
7 When the wine is completely clear, and fermentation has stopped, bottle, cork, and label. Store for six months before drinking.

Note

* Alternatively, in Step 1 coarsely grate the Marrow into the bin.

Parsnip
Pastinaca sativa

The taste of Parsnips is unlike that of any other vegetable, and much appreciated by those who like it, though it is not to all tastes. Parsnips are indigenous to Eurasia, where they are believed to have formed part of the diet since ancient times, and this edible and nutritious root is now a well-known vegetable in many parts of the world. Those who dislike the root itself may find themselves pleasantly surprised by the wine, which has been described as tasting like Madeira.

Parsnips are not found growing in the wild, so must be bought or grown at home. Most people will know the creamy white roots, swollen and tapering and with a strong, spicy scent. They demand a certain amount of dedication to be grown successfully, requiring deeply dug and well-drained loamy soil, on the limey side, and regular watering in dry weather because changing levels of moisture in the soil cause cracked roots.

Parsnips must be sown from fresh seed each year as the seeds soon lose their vigor. Seeds are sown in rows the previous winter or in early spring, and the young plants are thinned out when big enough to handle. The roots are harvested in late autumn and throughout the winter, those of best flavor being harvested after the frosts. They withstand the winter well, and can be left in the ground until required. Ease the roots out of the soil with a fork when you are ready.

Ocean voyage The Parsnip was introduced to North America by settlers from Britain, where it was already known and valued as a root vegetable. In the 1800s it lost favor as it was gradually supplanted by the potato.

Caution Some people are sensitive to the chemicals in Parsnip leaves and stems. As with hogweed, they can cause quite severe dermatitis in susceptible people, with a burning, blistering rash on skin that has been exposed. If affected, wash the skin immediately and keep out of sunlight, which aggravates the condition. In severe cases, seek medical advice. It would be a wise precaution to wear protective gloves when handling the plant.

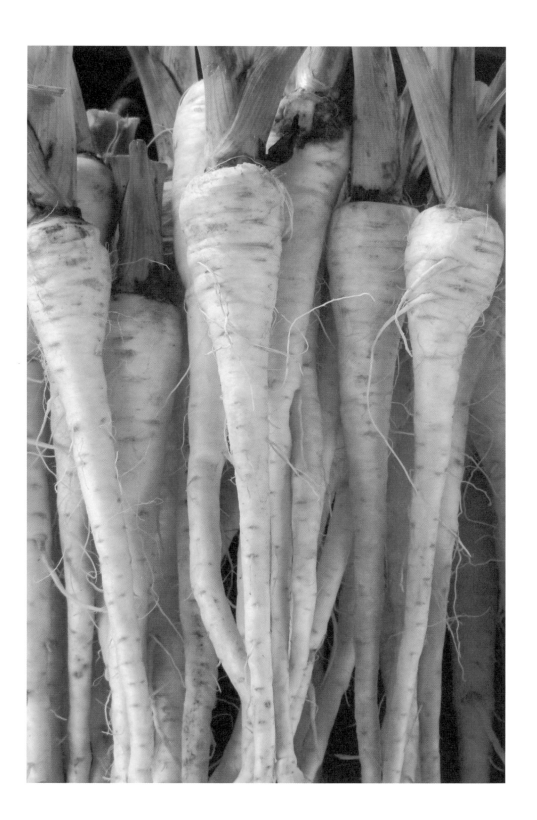

Parsnip Wine

Parsnips are at their sweetest after the frosts and traditionally this wine was made just after Christmas. Like Carrot Wine, it has a hint of Sherry about it and can be made with Sherry yeast. Slow maturing turns it into a tasty tipple.

You will need

* 1.8 kg (4 lb) old Parsnips
* 4.5 liters (1 gallon) water
* 1 lemon, scrubbed
* 1 Seville orange, scrubbed
* 1.3 kg (3 lb) sugar
* 225 g (8 oz) raisins, chopped
* 1 Campden tablet, crushed
* yeast and nutrient

Method

1   Wash and scrub the Parsnips and cut away any damaged or 'rusty' parts. Slice the roots into a preserving pan or large saucepan and boil them in the water until they are tender.
2   Thinly pare the lemon and orange and squeeze out the juice. Put the sugar, raisins, and pared zest into a fermenting bin and strain on the Parsnip liquid.
3   Stir well to dissolve the sugar, then add the fruit juice and the crushed Campden tablet. Stir, cover, and leave in a warm place for 24 hours.
4   Add the yeast, cover again, and leave to ferment for a week, stirring twice daily.
5   Strain off the liquid and transfer it to a demijohn, fit the airlock, and ferment in a warm place, racking as the sediment forms and the wine clears. (This may take six months.)
6   Bottle, cork, and label when fermentation is complete and the wine is clear (see Notes). Store for 18 months to mature.

Notes

* If possible, put the finished wine in a clean demijohn, put in a bung, and mature in the demijohn for six months before bottling, then store for at least a year.

* The cooked Parsnips left over from Step 1 can be used for soup, or simply eaten as normal.
* An old country version of this wine keeps fermentation going by adding a little more sugar to the demijohn from time to time to feed the yeast, so that a strong, sweet wine is produced.

Pea

Pisum sativum

also known as Garden Peas, English Peas, Green Peas

Garden Peas reached western Europe from northwest India in medieval times, but have not always been as popular as they are now. Peas now need no description and are enjoyed by almost everyone. It may even come as a surprise to some that they actually grow in pods, the frozen shelled Pea being so ubiquitous. Another 'vegetable' that has been on the menu since prehistory, Pea pods are technically a fruit, with the individual Peas being really the seeds. In fact, if you buy fresh Peas, or grow your own, the amount of wastage from the pods when the Peas have been shelled may seem shocking.

A climbing plant with clinging tendrils, Peas need something to climb up, in the form of twiggy sticks or pea netting secured on stakes. Depending on the variety, they can grow to a height of 1.5 m (5 ft), but many dwarf forms are available. The attractive creamy white flowers develop into the Pea pods from early summer, again depending on the variety selected.

Peas are quite easy to grow, given a cool climate, an open, sunny but sheltered position, and a moisture-retentive soil. They root deeply, so do best in a well and deeply dug plot, and they need a dressing of lime unless the soil is already limey, but in turn supply the soil with valuable nitrogen for crops that follow them. There is little waste in growing Peas, because the seeds can be sown individually. Pick the young pods off the plants regularly to encourage more.

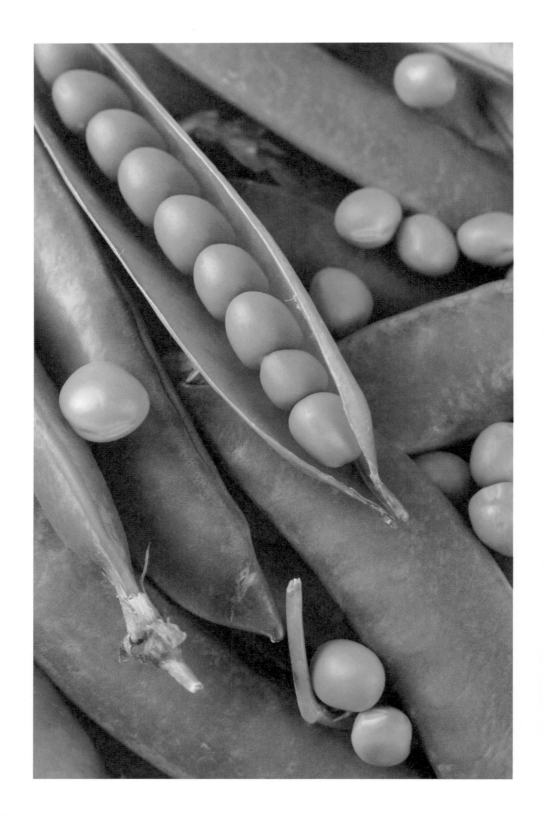

Green Peas Especially in old-fashioned cafés, garden Peas are referred to as 'Green Peas' on the menu. This dates back to the fact that for most of their 6,000- year-long history Peas were mainly left to become fully mature on the plant before being picked and used as a dried vegetable. Eating the fresh, immature Peas became a bit of a fashion fad in France and England in the 1700s and the seeds were distinguished by the name 'Green Peas.'

Transatlantic crop By the time of the Pilgrim Fathers, Peas had become a favorite English kitchen-garden crop, so naturally they were taken to be grown in the New World. Peas, fresh or dried, became equally popular in North America and eventually 30 different types of Pea were among the many plants cultivated by Thomas Jefferson on his estate in Virginia.

Pea Pod Wine

This is a very satisfying wine to make for anyone with a frugal approach to the kitchen. It uses fresh Pea Pods, which would otherwise be discarded or at best sent to the compost heap, and turns them into a clear white table wine.

You will need
* 1.8 kg (4 lb) Pea Pods
* 1 lemon, pared and squeezed
* 4.5 liters (1 gallon) water
* yeast and nutrient
* 1.3 kg (3 lb) sugar

Method
1 Boil the Pea Pods and lemon zest in a preserving pan or large saucepan, using all the water in the recipe.
2 Simmer for about 20 minutes, or until the Pea Pods are very tender. Activate the yeast during this time (see page 35).
3 Strain the liquid into a fermenting bin. Pour in the sugar and stir well, making sure the sugar is completely dissolved.
4 Add the lemon juice and allow the liquid to cool.
5 When the liquid is at blood heat, add in the yeast, cover, and leave to ferment for 24 hours, stirring once or twice.

6 Siphon into a demijohn, fit the airlock and leave to ferment in a warm place, racking as required.

7 When fermentation has ceased and the wine has cleared, bottle, cork, and label. Store for a minimum of six months.

Notes
* This is a very quick and simple wine to make, and one that should clear rapidly.
* Country people agree that the longer you can keep the wine the better it will taste.

Runner Bean
Phasiolus coccineus
also known as Runners, Scarlet Runners, String Bean

The Runner Bean originates in Central America, and was originally introduced to European gardens as an ornamental climbing plant, admired for its colorful red, pink, or white flowers. The beans themselves were at first of secondary interest, and early varieties such as 'Painted Lady' reflect this. Now, however, they are a much-loved crop in many vegetable gardens, though they are still also grown as ornamental plants in North America.

Runner Bean is a perennial (living on from year to year) but as a vegetable it is grown annually, and the plants do not withstand the winter temperatures of temperate regions. One of the reasons for the Beans' popularity is that they grow very quickly from a late spring or early summer sowing, to produce a plentiful crop of long green beans from late summer until the first cold weather.

To grow your own, sow the seed in late spring or early summer, preferably in trenches filled with garden compost or manure. Provide the support of stout poles and strong netting, as the plants are strong-growing, with large leaves, and they fruit heavily. They thrive on regular feeding and, like peas, need plenty of moisture. In dry weather, the flowers should be sprayed to help the fruit to set. For the kitchen you need to harvest the beans frequently, when they are young and tender and before they have grown long and coarse. Towards the end of the season, or after the summer holidays, you are bound to have some overgrown pods that have become tough and knobbly.

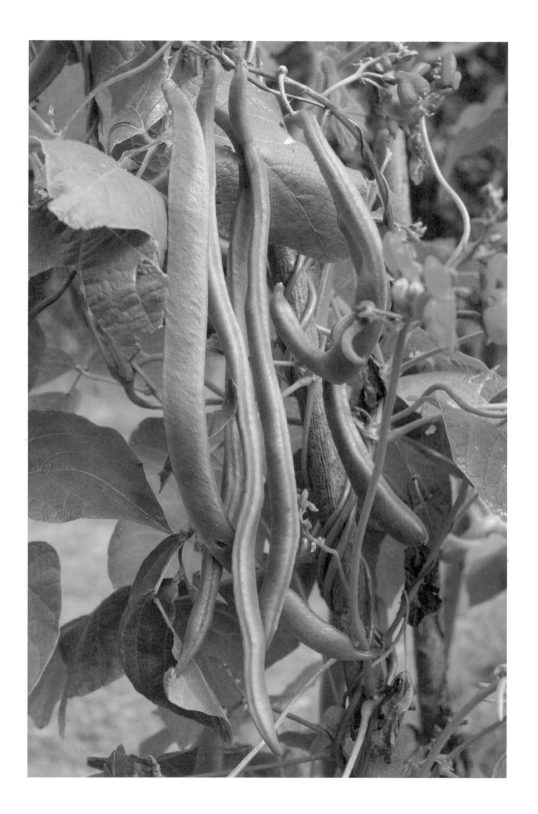

Runner Bean (String Bean) Wine

Making wine with Runner Beans is a perfect way of using up a surplus towards the end of the summer. It is worth experimenting at least once with this wine, which some liken to a crisp dry Sherry. To be fair, others say it tastes of Runner Beans – so try it and see.

You will need

* 1.3 kg (3 lb) Runner Beans
* 4.5 liters (1 gallon) water
* 340 g (12 oz) raisins, chopped
* 1.3 kg (3 lb) sugar
* 2.5 ml (½ teaspoon) grape tannin
* 1 lemon, squeezed
* yeast and nutrient

Method

1   Break the Beans into large pieces and boil them in the water until they are very well cooked.
2   Put the raisins and sugar into a fermenting bin and strain the cooking liquid onto them.
3   Add the grape tannin. Cover and allow to cool.
4   When the liquid has cooled to blood heat, add the lemon juice and yeast.
5   Cover and leave to ferment for a week, stirring daily, then strain off the liquid, transfer it to a demijohn and fit the airlock.
6   Leave in a warm place to ferment, racking as necessary. The wine should clear quite quickly.
7   When the wine is clear and fermentation has ceased, bottle, cork, and label. Store for at least a year.

Notes

* Large and rather stringy Runner Beans are fine, so the recipe will take care of those that have been left on the plant too long.
* Adding a banana skin or two can help to give body to the wine.
* For a more authentic country touch, use half a cup of cold tea instead of the grape tannin.
* Long keeping is crucial for this wine – the longer the better.

Swede
Brassica rutabaga
also known as Rutabaga, Swedish Turnip

Originating in Eurasia, Swedes are a root crop and were given their name on being introduced to Scotland from Sweden in the eighteenth century. Grown both as a vegetable and as cattle fodder, the round, firm roots are orange yellow inside, and the smooth surface is a dull orange, often purple at the top. Widely available throughout the year now, Swede should really be appreciated as a winter vegetable.

Turnip
Brassica rapa
also known as Neep

Like Swedes, Turnips are part of the Brassica family (which includes cabbages and cauliflowers) but are grown not for the leaves or heads but for the underground root. Much less sweet in flavor than the Swedes, Turnips come from the Mediterranean region and their round white or sometimes yellow roots have a slightly peppery taste. Most Turnips are globular in shape, though long-rooted varieties can be found.

Growing Swedes and Turnips While store-bought Swedes and Turnips are readily available during most of the year, they can both fairly easily be grown in the vegetable garden.

Swedes are best sown in late summer, which results in small but sweet and tasty winter vegetables. Any reasonably fertile soil will do, as long as it is not too acid, and as long as it has not been freshly manured, which causes the roots to fork. Like parsnips, Swedes need a regular and even supply of moisture and without it the roots may split. Also they can be left in the ground during the winter and dug up as required, though if the ground is frozen hard digging will not be possible.

The growing requirements for Turnips are similar to those of Swedes, but an earlier crop can also be grown in a sheltered position from a spring sowing. Young Turnips can be pulled out of the ground like radishes, while bigger, older ones should be dug up.

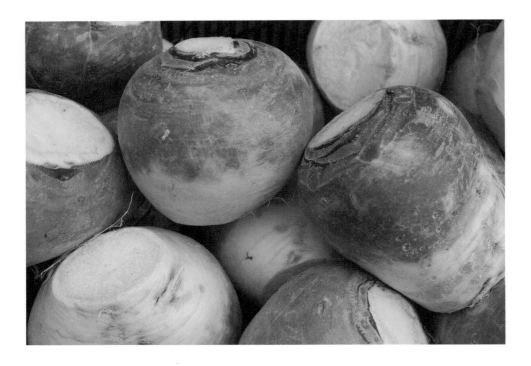

Swede Wine or Turnip Wine

Swedes and Turnips both make a surprisingly good wine, partly due to their sweetness. The same recipe will work for both roots, but you should omit the orange when making Turnip Wine. Swede Wine should be golden colored and Turnip Wine white.

You will need

* 1.8 kg (4 lb) Swedes (Rutabaga) or Turnips
* 4.5 liters (1 gallon) water
* 2 lemons, scrubbed
* 1 orange, scrubbed
* 1.3 kg (3 lb) sugar
* 225 g (8 oz) raisins, chopped
* 1 Campden tablet, crushed
* yeast and nutrient

Method

1 Wash and scrub the Swedes or Turnips and cut away any damaged or 'rusty' parts. Dice them and boil them in all the water in a preserving pan or large saucepan until they are soft and tender.

2 Thinly pare the lemons and orange and squeeze out the juice. Put the sugar, raisins, and pared zest into a fermenting bin and strain on the vegetable liquid.

3 Stir well to dissolve the sugar, then add the fruit juice and the crushed Campden tablet. Stir, cover, and leave in a warm place for 24 hours.

4 Add the yeast, cover again, and leave to ferment for about five days, stirring twice daily.

5 Strain off the liquid and transfer it to a demijohn, fit the airlock, and ferment in a warm place, racking as the sediment forms and the wine clears. (This may take six months.)

6 When fermentation has ceased and the wine is completely clear, bottle, cork, and label. Store for a year to mature.

Notes

∗ If the Swedes are very hard and difficult to cut, they can be softened in a microwave oven first. Put them in on a high setting for 20–60 seconds, depending on their size and hardness.

∗ The cooked Swedes or Turnips can be reserved in Step 2 to be used for soup or as a table vegetable.

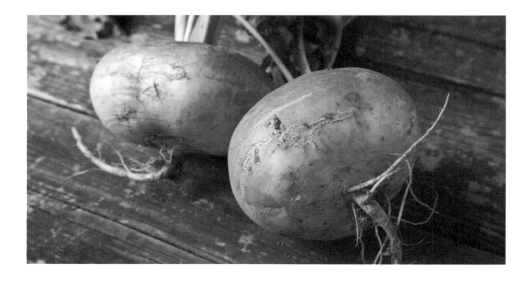

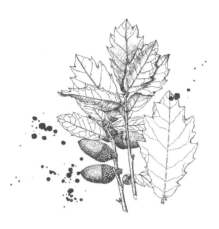

GRAIN, LEAF, AND STEM WINES

This final section is in some ways a bit of a rag-bag, encompassing ingredients that have long been used for traditional wines but that don't quite fit into the three main groups. Cereals like Barley contain much starch and import a strong flavor, but the starch can make winemaking tricky as the yeast has to work hard to break it all down. It is possible to obtain special cereal yeast, and beer yeast is sometimes used for cereals. Ginger wine is a good old favorite, so popular that is still made commercially. Rhubarb is another strong classic, and a well-made Rhubarb wine has much distinction. These three are still well known, but some of the other wines in this section, such as those made from leaves or herbs, are beginning to be forgotten and are now well worth trying for their novelty value, to keep them alive, and also because they make fine and unusual wines.

Barley

Hordeum **species**

also known as Pearl Barley, Scottish Barley

Barley is an ancient cereal crop that was vital to the development of civilization and is still a major crop worldwide today. Wild Barley was indigenous across a wide swathe of land from North Africa and Crete to Tibet. Archaeological remains show that it was domesticated in pre-pottery times and Barley Beer was probably the first alcoholic drink developed by our Neolithic ancestors.

What became know as Barley Wine is really an ale, being based on a malted grain. It was such a popular country drink that – like the pear drink, Perry – it was eventually made commercially on a large scale as more and more country people moved into cities. Barley water was a household remedy for all sorts of digestive complaints and a source of nourishment for the sick. It was also used as a soothing lotion for sore skin. Pearl Barley is the name given to the hulled Barley grain, which is used for making flour and Barley water.

What's in a name? Barley 'Wine' gets its name from the time of the Napoleonic wars. England was constantly at war with France, and the English felt obliged to deny themselves the pleasure of drinking French claret in favor of an English brew. The popular Barley ale they turned to was renamed 'Wine' in a sort of patriotic defiance.

The drink was indeed as strong as wine, and unlike beer had to be matured for 18–24 months. In grand English houses it was brewed by the butler and served from cut-glass goblets. Commercial brewing of the 'wine' began around 1870.

Barley Wine

This is a rich, full-flavored wine, which may well be rather strong, with a dark, fruity flavor. Drink it from small glasses as a dessert wine. This is one of the many traditional recipes that have potato and oranges among the ingredients.

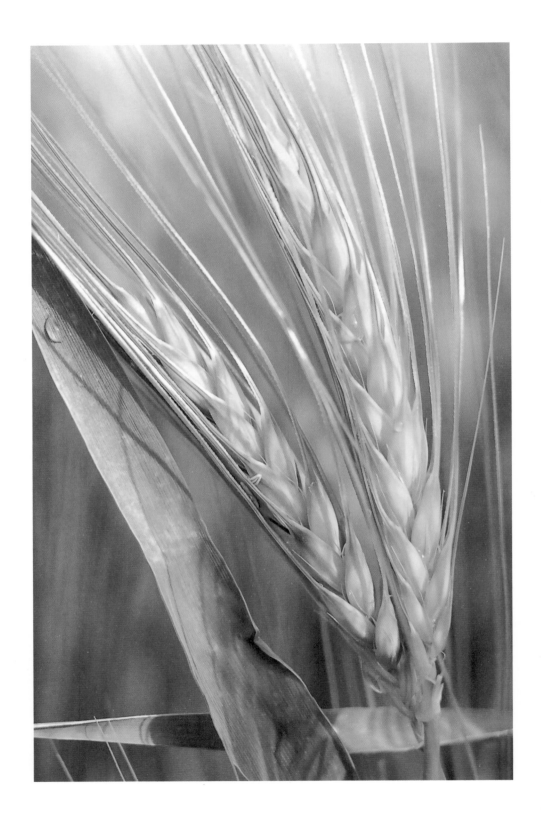

You will need

* 450 g (1 lb) pearl Barley
* 450 g (1 lb) raisins, chopped
* 1.3 kg (3 lb) Demerara sugar
* 2 old potatoes, scrubbed and sliced
* 1 orange, pared and squeezed
* 1 lemon, pared and squeezed
* 4.5 liters (1 gallon) water
* yeast and nutrient (see Note below)

Method

1 Put all the ingredients except the yeast and water into a fermenting bin and stir together.
2 Heat the water and when it is hot (but not boiling) pour it into the bin and stir it in.
3 Check the temperature, and add the yeast when the contents are at 21–24°C (70–75°F), or blood heat.
4 Cover and leave in a warm place to ferment.
5 Leave fermenting in the bin for ten days, stirring once or twice daily.
6 Strain off the liquid and transfer it to a demijohn. Fit the airlock and continue fermenting until bubbling has stopped and the wine is clear.
7 Move the jar to a cool place and keep it there for a few days before siphoning off the wine into bottles. Cork and label. Store for a year.

Note

* Cereal or brewers' yeast may be used.

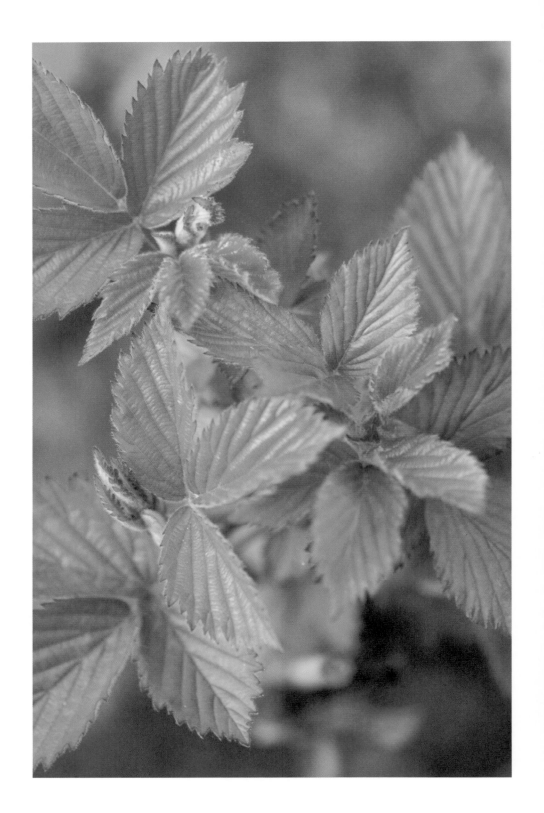

Blackberry Tip
Rubus fruticosus
also known as Bramble Tip
The Blackberry or Bramble plant is described under the recipes for Fruit Wines (see page 84). It is a wonderful wild resource for people who like to gather wine ingredients on country rambles. As the fruits are beginning to form during the summer, the plants are already preparing for the following year by putting out supple new canes, the tips of which are soft and tender. These are easy to pick and make an unusual but traditional country wine. Harvest the tips by picking off the tender part by hand. Scissors can be used if you wish, but even the prickles are less aggressive at this stage, so gloves are not vital. Put the Bramble Tips straight into a measuring bucket, or use a stout basket or canvas bag.

Blackberry Tip Wine
This is a low-cost wine that is simple to make and requires very little time to mature. The result should be a clear white table wine with a yellowish tint. It is best to judge the quantity of tips needed by volume rather than weight.

You will need
* 4.5 liters (1 gallon) of Bramble Tips (by volume)
* 4.5 liters (1 gallon) water
* 2 lemons, pared and squeezed
* 1.3 kg (3 lb) sugar
* 5 ml (1 teaspoon) acid blend (optional, see Method)
* yeast and nutrient

Method
1 Put the measured Bramble Tips in a colander that is standing in the sink, and rinse well to clean them. Tip them out into a preserving pan or large saucepan.
2 Pour the water over the Bramble Tips, add the pared lemon zest, bring to a boil, and simmer for about 20 minutes.
3 Put the sugar and lemon juice into a fermenting bin, then strain on the hot liquid from the Brambles. Stir well to dissolve the sugar and allow to cool to 21–24°C (70–75°F) or blood heat.
4 Add the acid blend if using this instead of lemon juice, and put in the yeast.

5   Cover and leave to ferment for two days, then transfer the liquid to a demijohn. Fit the airlock, then stand it in a warm place to continue fermenting. Tilt the jar occasionally to help the gases out while bubbling is fierce.

6   When fermentation slows and the wine is beginning to form a sediment, rack it into a clean demijohn. It should clear quite quickly after the first racking.

7   When bubbling stops, move it to a cooler place to allow the wine to clear in the dark.

8   When the wine is clear, siphon into bottles, cork, and label. Store for one year.

Note

*   When bubbling slows down in Step 6, you can add a little more sugar day by day (up to 225 g/8 oz in total) to allow the yeast to keep on working to make a stronger wine.

Ginger
Zingiber officinale

The household spice Ginger is the underground part of a tropical plant that is thought to originate from China and to have been transported into countries to the west over many centuries. Always a highly regarded spice in Europe, it was the first to be cultivated by Europeans in the New World, particularly in Jamaica, to meet the demand. Ginger soon caught on in North America, as indicated by the fact that it became part of the American revolutionary fighters' food rations. Even in recent times, Ginger jam was still *de rigueur* after high-class dinners in New England. We call it Ginger 'root,' but the part we use is really a rhizome or below-the-surface stem.

Ginger Beer and Ginger Wine are traditional popular drinks that used to be made in the home and became commercialized in the nineteenth century. While the beer is a cooling drink for summer, Ginger Wine is associated with winter and has warming effects. Whole fresh Ginger root is normally used, sliced or minced, according to the recipe.

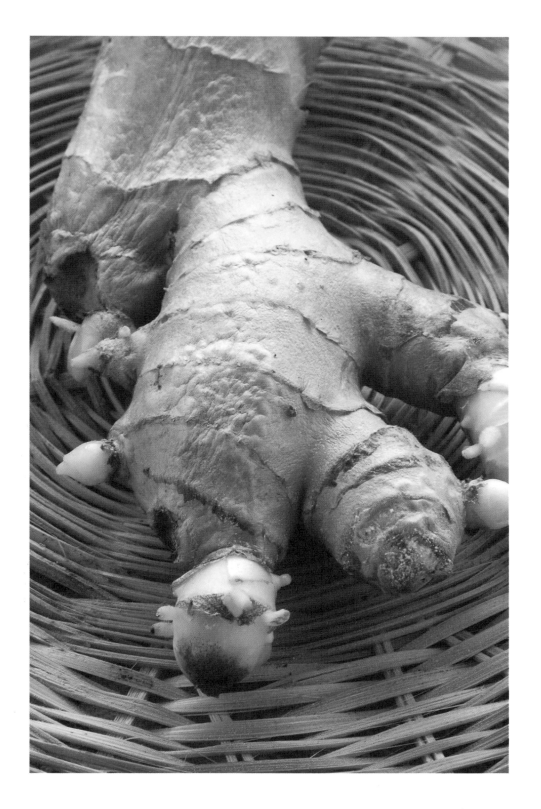

Old Ginger jars The Ancient Romans used Ginger that was imported to Rome from China and sold to them by Arabian traders in special little clay jars. The gullible Romans believed that the spice came from mysterious people who lived on the very edge of the Earth.

Ginger Wine

Ginger Wine is a traditional warming drink for Christmas, strong in both Ginger taste and alcohol, and served from little glasses – cut glass shows off its ginger biscuit color to perfection. Long storage is the key to success for this wine.

You will need

* 100 g (4 oz) Ginger root
* 450 g (1 lb) raisins, chopped
* 2 lemons, pared and squeezed
* 2 oranges, pared and squeezed
* 650 g (1½ lb) white sugar
* 450 g (1 lb) Demerara sugar
* 2 bananas or 5 ml (1 teaspoon) grape tannin
* 4.5 liters (1 gallon) water
* yeast and nutrient

1 Roughly crush or thinly slice the Ginger and put it into a fermenting bin with the raisins, zest and juice of the lemons and oranges, and all the sugar.
2 Chop the bananas, with their skins, and add them to the bin. Alternatively, use grape tannin.
3 Bring the water to a boil and pour it into the bin. Stir well until the sugar is completely dissolved. Cover and allow to cool to around 21°C (70°F), then add the yeast.
4 Leave in a warm place to ferment for a week, stirring frequently.
5 Strain the liquid off the solids and transfer it to a demijohn. Fit the airlock and leave in a warm place to continue fermenting. Rack as required, until the wine is clear.
6 Transfer the finished wine to a clean demijohn, put in a bung and store in a cool, dark place for six months. Bottle, cork, and label at the end of this period. Store the wine for a minimum of one more year before tasting.

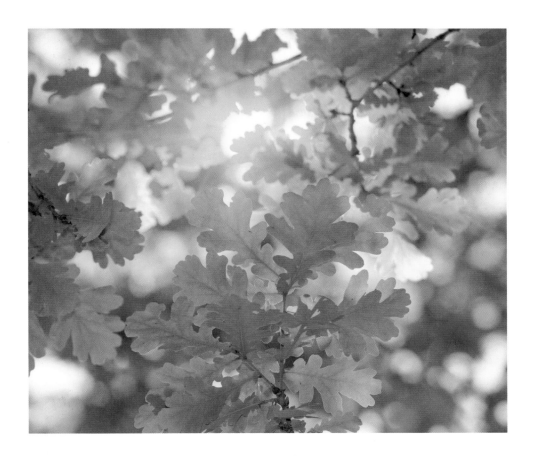

Oak

Quercus robur

also known as Common Oak, English Oak, Pedunculate Oak, Truffle Oak

A native tree in Europe, western Asia, and North Africa, the sturdy Oak has been planted in many other parts of the world, while several closely related forms are indigenous in various parts of the United States. A symbol of stability and reliability, Oak trees can live for hundreds of years. They form rugged, lofty, acorn-bearing trees that can be 25 m (80 ft) high, with broad trunks, spreading branches and bluntly lobed leaves. In early summer, the newly mature leaves can be used to make an interesting wine.

Leaf it alone Taking sap for wines is not recommended, as this can seriously harm the tree, but the spring and early-summer leaves of various trees can be used. Oak and Walnut are old country favorites.

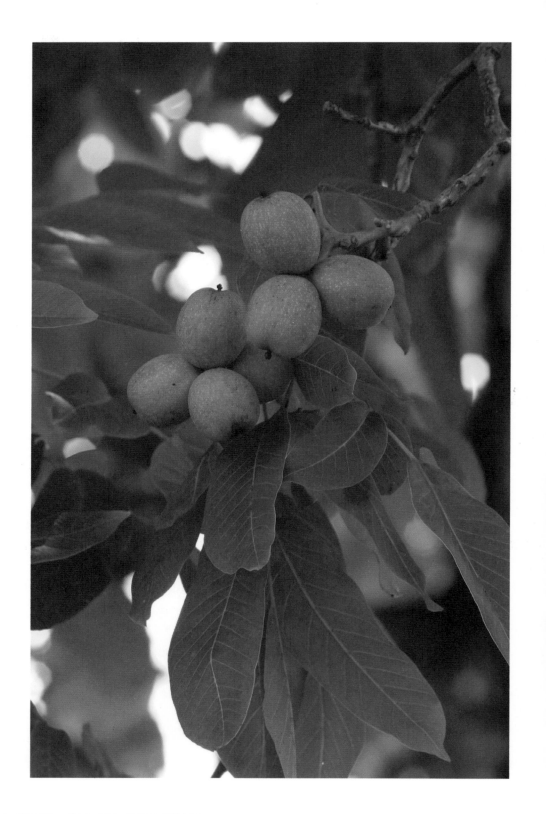

Walnut The Walnut, *Juglans regia* (Europe) and *Juglans nigra* (North America), is often found as an ornamental nut-producing tree of old established gardens – less frequently in the wild. A stately tree with grey bark, it bears the fruits protected by a thick and spongy, yellowish-green outer casing in late summer. The leaves consist of several paired leaflets, topped with a single leaflet, and in spring they can be used to make Walnut Leaf Wine, following the recipe for Oak Leaf.

Oak Leaf or Walnut Leaf Wine

You will need
* 2.3 liters (4 pints) Oak leaves or 1 large handful new Walnut Leaves
* 4.5 liters (1 gallon) water
* 1.3 kg (3 lb) sugar
* 2 lemons, pared and squeezed
* 2 oranges, pared and squeezed
* 225 g (8 oz) raisins, chopped
* yeast and nutrient

Method
1   Rinse the leaves to clean them, then put them into a large container. Bring the water to a boil and pour it over the leaves.
2   Cover and leave to infuse for 24 hours.
3   Put the sugar into a fermenting bin with the pared zest and the chopped raisins. Strain off the infusion into a large pan and heat it up to about 24°C (75°F).
4   Pour the infusion into the bin, and stir well to dissolve the sugar. Allow it to cool a little, then add the citrus fruit juices and the yeast. Cover and leave in a warm place to ferment, stirring daily.
5   After four or five days, strain off the liquid and transfer it to a demijohn. Fit the airlock and leave in a warm place for fermentation to continue, racking once or twice as the sediment forms.
6   When fermentation has ceased and the wine is clear, bottle, cork, and label. Store for six months.

Parsley

Petroselinum crispum

Parsley is native to the central Mediterranean region (particularly southern Italy, Sardinia, and parts of north Africa), but the herb is cultivated much more widely and has become naturalized in some parts of Europe. Despite its sunny origins, it enjoys a well-drained but moist soil and needs to be watered in dry weather. It will grow in partial shade as long as it is in a warm, well-sheltered place.

Every kitchen garden or allotment should have its own supply of Parsley. In flower gardens, the herb makes a good edging plant. For a continuous supply, sow the seeds outdoors three times a year: in late winter, mid-spring, and again in late summer. Sow them directly in shallow drills in well-prepared ground or start them off in a seed-box. Seeds can be slow to germinate, and one way to encourage them is to pour warm water gently over the seedbed or seed-box immediately after sowing. Don't be in a hurry to see the first green leaves appearing.

During the summer, growth can be coarse, and to encourage fresh new growth it is advisable to cut off all the leaves. This is the time to make your Parsley Wine, using the cut-off leaves and stems.

Country lore Where Parsley flourishes, the woman wears the trousers.

Caution Though Parsley can be found growing wild, there are many other plants it can be confused with. These include the poisonous Fool's Parsley and deadly Hemlock. Always use Parsley grown specifically for kitchen use in a garden or allotment (or from the greengrocers) and never try to pick it in the wild.

Attracting wildlife If you have a large crop of Parsley, allow some of it to flower and run to seed. The flowers will attract bees and hoverflies to the garden, and the seeds provide food for goldfinches and other seed-loving birds.

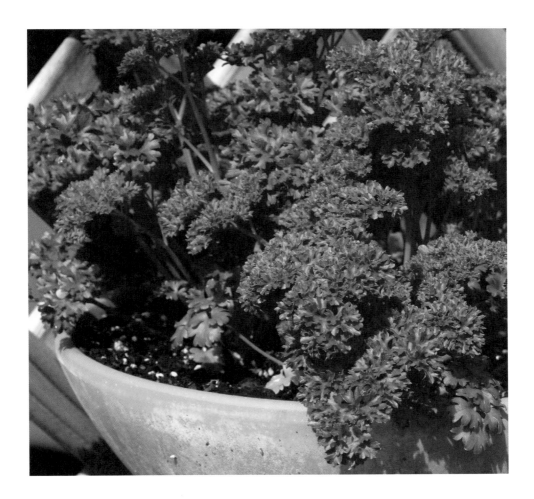

Parsley Wine

Use outdoor-grown Parsley to make wine, not the flimsy Parsley sold in pots in supermarkets as this is not nearly sturdy enough. The recipe should make a fine white wine that slightly resembles Hock. A Hock yeast can be used to help achieve this effect.

You will need

* 225 g (8 oz) Parsley
* 1 lemon, pared and squeezed
* 4.5 liters (1 gallon) water
* 1.2 kg (2½ lb) sugar
* 225 g (8 oz) sultanas, chopped
* yeast and nutrient (see above)

Method

1 Simmer the Parsley and lemon zest in the water for 20 minutes.
2 Put the sugar and sultanas into a fermenting bin and strain the hot liquid over them. Stir well to dissolve the sugar.
3 Cool the syrup to blood heat (21–24°C/70–75°F), then add the lemon juice and yeast.
4 Cover and leave in a warm place to ferment, stirring twice daily.
5 Strain off the liquid and transfer it to a demijohn, fit the airlock, and leave in a warm place to continue fermenting, racking as required.
6 When all bubbling has ceased and the wine is clear, bottle, cork, and label. Store for six months.

Rhubarb

Rheum rhaponticum, **also known as** *Rheum × cultorum*

A well-tended Rhubarb plant can thrive for 20 years and will provide quantities of succulent stems each year from early summer. The stems are yellowy-green to pinkish-red, with enormous dark green leaves. Only the stems themselves are edible, known for their tart, acid flavor. The plant will grow to 60 cm (2 ft) high and may develop to a spread of 2 m (6 ft) over its long life.

Rhubarb will grow in any well-drained garden soil, but rewards attention. The ground should be given well-rotted manure or garden compost in the autumn and a dose of fertilizer in spring. It should also be kept free of weeds. Flowering stems should be removed as they appear to encourage continued growth of the edible stems (known as 'sticks'). Give the plants a good mulching early in the year to keep the earth moist, and water them in dry weather.

Rhubarb can be harvested from its second year. Hold single stems firmly at the base and give a twist, pulling them away from the plant.

Caution It is only the Rhubarb stems themselves that are edible: the impressive leaves contain oxalic acid, and are poisonous.

Gardener's Tip 'Hawke's Champagne' is an early Rhubarb variety, with deep red stems. A good cropper, it seems to be asking to be made into sparkling wine.

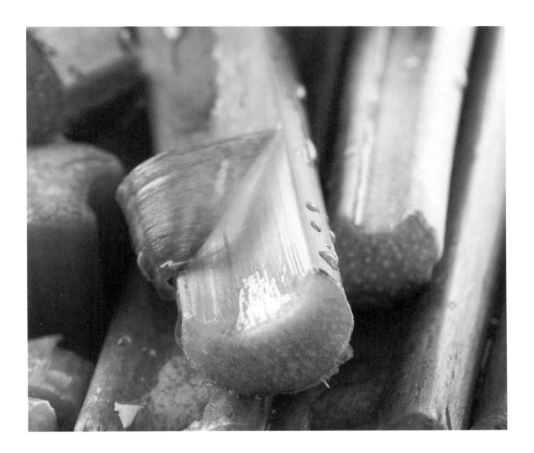

Rhubarb Wine

Rhubarb makes an attractive blush-colored wine that should be fairly dry, and minimal preparation is involved in making it. Tender stems are best for pies and other desserts, but the coarser, more mature ones are perfect for Rhubarb Wine.

You will need
* 1.3 kg (3 lb) Rhubarb
* 1.3 kg (3 lb) sugar
* 225 g (8 oz) sultanas, chopped
* 1 lemon, scrubbed and pared
* 1 Campden tablet, crushed
* 4.5 liters (1 gallon) water
* yeast and nutrient
* 1 vitamin C tablet, crushed

Method

1 Wipe the Rhubarb clean, cut the sticks into pieces (no need to string them), and place it all in a large container or fermenting bin.

2 Pour the sugar over the chopped-up Rhubarb, add the chopped sultanas, lemon zest, and crushed Campden tablet, stir, and cover.

3 Leave for 24 hours, then add the yeast. Heat up the water to 21°C (70°F) and pour it over the mixture. Cover and leave to ferment for two days only, stirring twice daily.

4 Strain the liquid off the pulp, pressing to extract it all, and transfer it to a fermenting bin. Cover and leave it in a warm place for another three or four days to ferment vigorously.

5 Transfer the liquid to a demijohn, fit the airlock, and leave in a warm place to continue fermenting. Rack the wine as it clears (this should be after about three weeks and again up to three months later).

6 When fermentation has stopped and the wine is clear, add a crushed vitamin C tablet to prevent oxidation, and siphon it into bottles. Cork and label. Store for at least six months.

Sparkling Rhubarb Wine

To make a sparkling wine, follow the recipe for Rhubarb Wine, but bottle the wine in strong, Champagne-type bottles in Step 6 and add a small teaspoon of sugar to each bottle. Use purpose-made plastic stoppers and wire them firmly in place. Store the bottles upright in a cool, dark place for six months to a year, checking occasionally that the stoppers are holding firm. Don't worry about the slight sediment that forms at the base of the bottles.

INDEX

Acknowledgements

Photographs: Fine Folio Publishing, Fotolia, iStockphoto and Photos.com.
Special thanks to Richard Cumming of Orchard Park (www.orchardpark.biz)
for supplying the Mangel Wurzel picture on page 158.